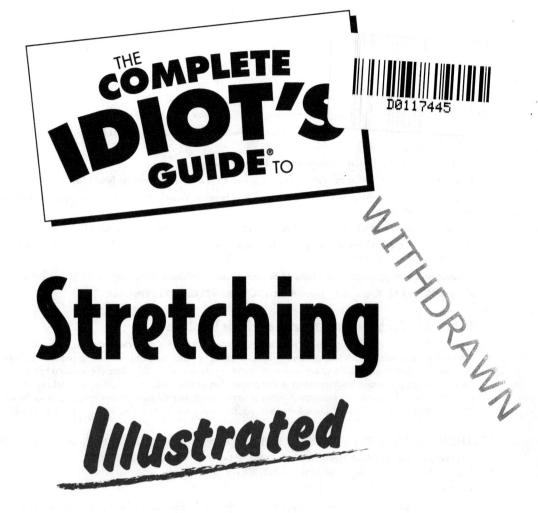

# THE COMPLETE IDIOT'S GUIDE® TO

# Stretching

## Illustrated

*by Barbara Templeton and Jamie Templeton*

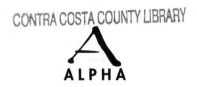

## ALPHA

A member of Penguin Group (USA) Inc.

## ALPHA BOOKS

Published by the Penguin Group

Penguin Group (USA) Inc., 375 Hudson Street, New York, New York 10014, USA

Penguin Group (Canada), 90 Eglinton Avenue East, Suite 700, Toronto, Ontario M4P 2Y3, Canada (a division of Pearson Penguin Canada Inc.)

Penguin Books Ltd., 80 Strand, London WC2R 0RL, England

Penguin Ireland, 25 St. Stephen's Green, Dublin 2, Ireland (a division of Penguin Books Ltd.)

Penguin Group (Australia), 250 Camberwell Road, Camberwell, Victoria 3124, Australia (a division of Pearson Australia Group Pty. Ltd.)

Penguin Books India Pvt. Ltd., 11 Community Centre, Panchsheel Park, New Delhi—110 017, India

Penguin Group (NZ), 67 Apollo Drive, Rosedale, North Shore, Auckland 1311, New Zealand (a division of Pearson New Zealand Ltd.)

Penguin Books (South Africa) (Pty.) Ltd., 24 Sturdee Avenue, Rosebank, Johannesburg 2196, South Africa

Penguin Books Ltd., Registered Offices: 80 Strand, London WC2R 0RL, England

## Copyright © 2007 by Barbara Templeton and Jamie Templeton

International Standard Book Number: 978-1-59257-621-0
Library of Congress Catalog Card Number: 2007928979

09  08  07    8  7  6  5  4  3  2  1

Interpretation of the printing code: The rightmost number of the first series of numbers is the year of the book's printing; the rightmost number of the second series of numbers is the number of the book's printing. For example, a printing code of 07-1 shows that the first printing occurred in 2007.

*Printed in the United States of America*

**Publisher:** *Marie Butler-Knight*
**Editorial Director:** *Mike Sanders*
**Managing Editor:** *Billy Fields*
**Senior Acquisitions Editor:** *Paul Dinas*
**Senior Development Editor:** *Christy Wagner*
**Production Editor:** *Megan Douglass*
**Copy Editor:** *Krista Hansing Editorial Services, Inc.*

**Cartoonist:** *Richard King*
**Cover Designer:** *Bill Thomas*
**Book Designer:** *Trina Wurst*
**Indexer:** *Julie Bess*
**Layout:** *Chad Dressler*
**Proofreader:** *Mary Hunt*

# Contents at a Glance

**Part 1:**    **The Anatomy of Stretching**    **2**

   1   Life's a Stretch    4
*Stretching improves the quality of your life by contracting and
releasing your muscles to lengthen, strengthen, and lubricate them.*

   2   Stretching Basics    10
*Ease your way into your stretching routine with these fundamental
mind and body warm-ups, and soon you'll find stretching is a healthy
habit you want to make time for.*

**Part 2:**    **Stretching from Head to Toe**    **22**

   3   Opening the Top of Your Body    24
*If you hold a lot of tension in your upper body, the stretches in this
chapter will leave you feeling like you just had a relaxing massage.*

   4   Hips, Legs, Thighs, and Feet—Your Base    40
*Strengthen your base to help keep you upright and stable—or set
you in motion.*

   5   Stretching Your Whole Body    62
*The simple stretching routines in this chapter take care of "the whole
enchilada."*

**Part 3:**    **Niche Stretching: Customizing Your Routine**    **80**

   6   Relieving Head, Neck, and Shoulder Discomfort    82
*Bring fast relief to tightness or soreness in these parts of your body
prone to mental and emotional stress.*

   7   Easing Joint Pain and Stiffness    94
*Relieve arthritis symptoms, post-workout joint aches, and early
morning stiffness with these easy stretches.*

   8   Sore Backs Stop Here    106
*Listen carefully to your back's aches and pains, and give it the
attention and care it deserves with the soothing stretches in this chapter.*

   9   Sports Stretching    122
*No matter what you play or how you play it, stretch to keep at the
top of your game.*

   10   Seniors' Stretch    150
*Reduce the chances of illness and injury as you age by maintaining
strength, flexibility, and balance.*

11  Just for Her                                                            158
    *Pamper yourself with these routines designed for women to experience*
    *their unique stages of life with grace.*

## Appendixes

    A  Glossary                                                             181
    B  Program Appendix                                                     185
    C  Stretching Resources                                                211
    D  Find Out More                                                        213
       Index                                                                215

# Contents

**Part 1:**  The Anatomy of Stretching                                          2

   **1**  Life's a Stretch ...................................................................4

      What Is Stretching? ..........................................................5

      Stretching Is Beneficial for Your Body ...........................6

         *Stretching—a Healthful Habit* ..................................6

         *Stretch to Heal* ...........................................................7

         *Stretching Keeps You Aligned and in Balance* ...........7

      Anyone Can Stretch ...........................................................8

      A Note of Caution Before You Start ................................9

   **2**  Stretching Basics ...........................................................10

      Anatomy of Elasticity .....................................................11

      Your Stretching Ritual ....................................................12

      Mindful Stretching ..........................................................13

      Dynamic and Static Stretching .......................................13

      PNF Stretching ................................................................14

      Breathing Into Your Stretch ...........................................14

      Listening to Your Body ....................................................15

      Warming Up .....................................................................16

         *Morning Stretch* .......................................................17

         *Bicycling* ...................................................................17

         *Gentle Twist* ..............................................................18

         *Spinal Roll* ...............................................................19

         *Hamstring Stretch* .....................................................20

**Part 2:**  Stretching from Head to Toe                                        22

   **3**  Opening the Top of Your Body .......................................24

      The Head Leads the Way .................................................26

         *Eagle Eye Stretch* .....................................................26

         *Eye Push-Ups* ...........................................................28

         *Jolly Jaws* .................................................................29

      Upper Back, Shoulders, and Chest ................................30

         *Sun and Earth* ..........................................................30

         *Pretzel* ......................................................................32

         *Figure Eight* .............................................................33

         *Relaxing Chest Opener* ............................................34

         *Chest Expander* ........................................................34

         *Prayer* ......................................................................36

Wrists and Hands.................................................................37
  *Finger Wrap*...................................................................37
  *Wrist Waves*..................................................................38
  *Wrist Circles*..................................................................38

4    Hips, Legs, Thighs, and Feet—Your Base ................40
  Base Basics.......................................................................41
  Hip Openers.....................................................................42
    *Diamond*........................................................................42
    *Number 4* .....................................................................43
    *Runner's Stretch*..........................................................45
    *Reclining Hip Flexor Stretch* ......................................46
    *Standing Hip Flexor Stretch* .......................................46
  Stretching Your Legs .......................................................48
    *Pyramid*........................................................................49
    *Kneeling Quadriceps Stretch* ......................................50
    *Standing Quadriceps Stretch*.......................................51
    *Hamstring Stretch with Hands*....................................52
    *Inner Thigh Stretch*......................................................54
    *Outer Thigh Stretch*.....................................................55
  Fabulous Feet, Knees, and Calves....................................56
    *On Your Toes*.................................................................56
    *Toe Tingler*....................................................................57
    *Ankles Alive*..................................................................58
    *Ankle Circles*.................................................................59
    *Double Knee Bends*......................................................60

5    Stretching Your Whole Body .....................................62
  Gentle Stretches................................................................64
    *Receiving Stretch*..........................................................64
    *Gentle Side Stretch*.......................................................65
    *Gentle Twist*..................................................................67
    *Gentle Half Back Stretch*..............................................68
    *Gentle Full Back Stretch* ..............................................70
  Strong Stretches................................................................71
    *Shoulder and Chest Expander*......................................71
    *Strong Side Stretch* .......................................................73
    *Strong Twist* ..................................................................74
    *Strong Half Back Stretch*..............................................76
    *Strong Full Back Stretch* ..............................................77

**Part 3:   Niche Stretching: Customizing Your Routine                        80**

6   Relieving Head, Neck, and Shoulder Discomfort.........................82
  Reverse Gravity to Cure Headaches ........................................84
    *Heels Over Head Stretch* ...................................................84
    *A Frame Stretch* .............................................................85
  Temporomandibular Joint Disorder (TMJD)...........................87
    *Deep Breathing*..............................................................87
    *Relax Your Jaw* .............................................................88
    *Stretch Your Jaw* ...........................................................88
  Nursing Your Neck.................................................................89
    *Seated Neck Stretch*........................................................89
    *Kneeling Neck Stretch* ....................................................90
  Stretching Sore Shoulders .....................................................91
    *Supine Shoulder Stretch* .................................................92
    *Sun and Earth* ...............................................................93

7   Easing Joint Pain and Stiffness...............................................94
  Carpal Tunnel Syndrome ......................................................96
    *Entire Front Stretch*........................................................96
    *Pretzel* ..........................................................................97
    *Reclining Fork* ...............................................................99
    *Bowl*.............................................................................100
  Hip and Knee Remedies ........................................................101
    *Single Knee Bends*..........................................................101
    *Reclining Hip Flexor Stretch* ..........................................102
    *Triangle Stretch* .............................................................103
    *Outer Thigh Stretch*........................................................104

8   Sore Backs Stop Here .............................................................106
  Essential Ways to Treat a Sore Back.......................................108
    *Relax Your Back on the Ball*............................................108
    *Arch and Curl*.................................................................109
    *Knee Press*.....................................................................110
    *Z Stretch*........................................................................111
    *Knee as Handle* ..............................................................112
    *Heels Over Head Stretch* ..................................................113
  Dealing With Sciatica.............................................................114
    *Seated Sciatic Stretch*......................................................114
    *One Leg Up, One Leg Down* ............................................115
    *Reclining Right Angle* .....................................................116
    *Standing Right Angle* ......................................................116
    *Outer Thigh Stretch*........................................................118

Back Strengtheners ..................................................................119

*Spinal Roll* ..............................................................................*119*

*Reclining Fork* .........................................................................*120*

*Dragon's Tail* ..........................................................................*121*

9    Sports Stretching ............................................................122

Sports Stretching Basics ........................................................124

Walking, Running, and Hiking ............................................124

*Pyramid* ...................................................................................*125*

*One Leg Up, One Leg Down* ...................................................*127*

*Kneeling Hip Flexor Stretch* ..................................................*128*

*Standing Quadriceps Stretch* .................................................*129*

*Triangle Stretch with Moving Leg* .........................................*130*

Cycling ......................................................................................131

*Z Stretch* ..................................................................................*132*

*Asymmetrical Hip Stretch* ......................................................*133*

Swimming .................................................................................134

*A Frame Stretch* ......................................................................*134*

*Diamond* ..................................................................................*136*

*Ankles Alive* ............................................................................*136*

*Pretzel* ......................................................................................*138*

Golf and Tennis .......................................................................139

*Wrist Waves* .............................................................................*139*

*Seated Neck Stretch* ................................................................*140*

*Ankle Circles* ...........................................................................*141*

*Reclining Twist* ........................................................................*142*

*Standing Squat* ........................................................................*143*

*Puppy Stretch* ..........................................................................*144*

*Standing Quadriceps Stretch* .................................................*145*

*Knee Press* ...............................................................................*146*

*Standing Chest Stretch* ...........................................................*147*

*Lunging Forward and Back* ....................................................*148*

10    Seniors' Stretch ..............................................................150

Sit and Stretch ........................................................................152

*Seated Chest Expander* ...........................................................*152*

*Seated Twist* ............................................................................*154*

*Seated Forward Bend* ..............................................................*155*

Standing Your Ground ..........................................................156

*Standing Balance Exercise: Part 1* ........................................*156*

*Standing Balance Exercise: Part 2* ........................................*157*

11    Just for Her ..................................................................158
      PMS.....................................................................160
          *A Frame Stretch* ........................................................*160*
          *Leap Frog* ...............................................................*162*
          *Reclining Number 4 Stretch* .............................................*163*
      Pregnancy............................................................164
          *Reclining Frog*...........................................................*164*
          *Modified Twist* ..........................................................*165*
          *Right Angle at Wall* .....................................................*167*
          *Partner Squat*...........................................................*168*
          *Meditative Stretch*.......................................................*169*
          *Ankle Rolls*..............................................................*170*
      Menopause ..........................................................171
          *Back Arch* ...............................................................*171*
          *Knee Press*...............................................................*172*
          *Heels Over Head Stretch* .................................................*174*
          *J Stretch* ................................................................*175*
      Mindful Stretching for Stress Relief ..............................176
          *Z Stretch*................................................................*176*
          *Reclining Diamond*.......................................................*178*
          *Reclining Twist*..........................................................*179*

**Appendixes**

    A    Glossary......................................................................181

    B    Program Appendix .........................................................185

    C    Stretching Resources........................................................211

    D    Find Out More .............................................................213

         Index.........................................................................215

# Introduction

People stretch for different reasons. Most seek a way to become flexible and strong. Others want to stay limber and healthy. Many know that stretching enhances their ability to participate in their favorite sport or activity. Some need to relieve discomfort or pain. Whatever your reasons for starting a stretching routine, *The Complete Idiot's Guide to Stretching Illustrated* can assist you in accomplishing all your goals.

Use this book as your guide, proceeding step by step or focusing on a particular part of your body. In these pages, you'll find detailed instructions, illustrations, and timed routines that make stretching simple and easy to fit into your daily schedule.

Once you start, stretching will become a part of your life. You'll soon forget about those aches and pains and stretch because it feels good. It's time to get started and let stretching work its magic!

## How to Use This Book

This book is divided into three parts, moving from basic stretching routines to programs designed to meet your unique needs:

**Part 1, "The Anatomy of Stretching,"** provides you with basic stretching concepts and techniques.

**Part 2, "Stretching from Head to Toe,"** teaches you how to stretch, starting at the top of your body, moving downward, and finally ending with whole body routines.

**Part 3, "Niche Stretching: Customizing Your Routine,"** offers customized stretching routines to meet your specific, personal needs.

## Stretch Maximizers

Throughout this book, you can *s-t-r-e-t-c-h* more deeply by investigating the bonus information housed in these boxes:

**Flexicon** _____
These boxes provide definitions of terms that assist you in understanding the process and benefits of stretching your body.

**Flex Alert!** _____
These cautionary boxes highlight information to assist you in safe stretching.

**S-t-r-e-t-c-h It Out** _____
These boxes contain tips and insights that help you get the best out of each stretch.

**A Stretch in Time ...** _____
These boxes offer you time-saving tips that help make stretching part of your daily routine.

## Acknowledgments

This book is dedicated to my husband, Jamie, my lifelong best friend. You make my dreams come true.

I offer my gratitude to the following people who made my book possible: to my friend, Cyndi Carr, and my literary agent, Andrea Hurst, for unexpectedly answering a lifelong prayer; to my daughter, Wray, for the joy you bring to my life; to my first teachers, my parents, Edward and Teresa Tomaszek, for my life and for your love, support, and encouragement; to Swami Kripalu and all the teachers at the Kripalu Center for Yoga and Health, for giving me my strong foundation in yoga; to Yogacharya Shri T. Krishnamacharya, the foremost modern yoga master known as the teacher of our teachers; to my beloved teachers, Srivatsa Ramaswami and Mark Whitwell, for teaching me how to breathe, providing me with my personal practice, and most of all for your love; to teachers Sara Mata, Sylvia Boorstein, Jack Kornfield, Ted Surman, Johnna Trimmer, and Annabel Raab, for your guidance, wisdom, generosity, and kindness; to all of my yoga students, who have taught me more than they will ever know; to Paul Dinas, my acquisitions editor at Alpha Books, for his support and expertise; to Jim Moran, my editor and writing mentor; to Craig Lockwood; to my friend and role model, Megan McDonough, for teaching me how to say "yes"; to Rob Talbert, for helping me stay healthy; to kind friends Manny, Jane, Sara, Summer, Diana, Jenny, Glynis, and Ann, for listening; and finally, to fellow teachers Trish Deignan and Jennifer Legault, for your expert contributions.

## Trademarks

# In This Part

1  Life's a Stretch

2  Stretching Basics

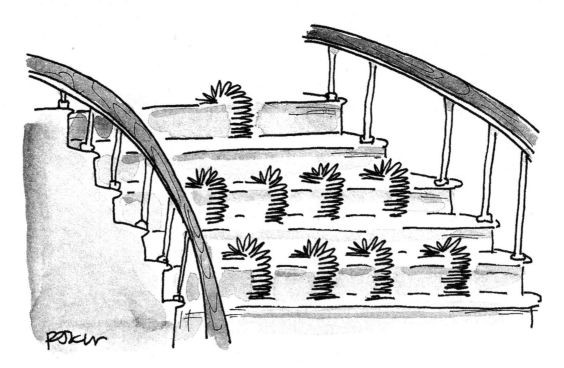

*"That's it, hold it, feel it, and six and seven…"*

# The Anatomy of Stretching

Part 1 provides you with basic stretching concepts and techniques. Here you discover what it means to stretch your body. Stretching as a means of maintaining a strong, healthy, and flexible body is explained, as well as the countless benefits of a daily stretching program. And now that you're motivated to stretch, you take a quick course in Anatomy 101 before exploring key stretching styles and breathing fundamentals. Then it's time to start your daily routine by practicing a few basic warm-ups.

## In This Chapter

- ◆ Stretching defined
- ◆ Understanding how stretching helps keep you healthy, flexible, strong, and balanced
- ◆ Healing your body with stretching
- ◆ Even *you* can stretch!

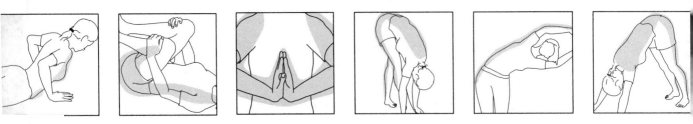

# Chapter 1

# Life's a Stretch

Stretching isn't anything new—it's actually one of your natural impulses. Think about it for a moment. You've been stretching all your life. We stretch as we come into the world as babies, as we grow into awkward adolescents, and as we mature as adults. We stretch before we get out of bed in the morning and when we take a warm, soothing shower. We stretch after sitting at our desks. The animals in our life even know the benefits of stretching—how many times have you seen your dog or cat wake up from a restful nap with a big stretch? We stretch because it feels good.

During the course of our daily lives, however, we seldom focus on our bodies. Feeling pressure and suffering stress, we take the weight of the world on our shoulders. Our mental and physical armor creates rigid bodies that diminish, if not downright ignore, our urge to stretch.

Theoretically, though, there's no reason why we can't be as flexible as babies. Stretching is the way to rediscover that youthful feeling, to make our bodies move naturally, even playfully. So why not give it a try? You might be surprised at how easy it is to make stretching a healthful habit.

## What Is Stretching?

If you've ever watched a child or even a cat or dog stretch, you'll learn a great deal about your need to stretch. *Stretching* is an integral part of human life and nature. You were made to twist, bend, and be in motion. Flexibility is both functional and pleasurable.

> **Flexicon** _____
>
> **Stretching** is the activity of contracting and releasing muscles to lengthen, strengthen, and lubricate them.

Every stretch is a marriage of effort and release. Stretching automatically contracts your muscles. In turn, contracted muscles cause other muscles to lengthen and extend. This union of "push and pull" creates strength and flexibility.

Take, for instance, the way your body feels after spending time in one position. It eventually knows it needs to stretch. When you let your body be your guide, you'll create a stretching routine that feels natural, not forced. And before you know it, you'll feel lighter, reach more easily, and move freely.

# Stretching Is Beneficial for Your Body

You'll welcome the benefits regular stretching brings. Daily tasks such as bending forward to tie your shoes or rushing to catch a bus become less strenuous as you increase your flexibility and _range of motion_. Flexibility, coordination, and balance tend to diminish as you age, but stretching can recover and preserve these qualities. As your body moves freely, you'll maintain coordination and balance, which will keep you mobile and less prone to injuries caused by falling.

> **Flexicon** _____
>
> **Range of motion** is a measurement of movement through a particular joint's or muscle's range.

Stretching helps our bodies "go with the flow" by balancing and providing appropriate tone and suppleness to our muscles. But that's just the beginning! Stretching causes a chain reaction (a good one!) in your muscles and throughout your body:

- With weak muscles strengthened and tight muscles lengthened, your posture improves.
- Standing tall minimizes discomfort and helps reduce common aches and pains.
- Circulation increases, providing a fresh supply of blood to rejuvenate, cleanse, and nourish your body.
- Recovery time from muscle injuries is shortened as toxins are released.

Most important, stretching loosens up tense muscles that habitually accompany stress. And as your muscles release …

- You relax.
- You sleep peacefully.
- You feel more at ease as tensions fade.
- You feel vital!

Let's face it—on top of all the other important and beneficial things stretching does, it just makes you feel _good!_

## Stretching—a Healthful Habit

"I'm really bad about stretching."

"I don't have time to stretch."

"I'm careful when I work out, so I don't need to stretch."

Do any of these comments sound like something you've thought or said? Even if these thoughts have crossed your mind or your lips, don't let them keep you from enjoying the benefits of stretching.

Choosing to stretch is no different from choosing to eat more fresh fruit and vegetables. It's never too late or too difficult to become active and take care of your body. Decide now to make stretching part of your life—you're worth it! Right now is the best time to start gaining the health benefits of a regular stretching routine.

### A Stretch in Time ...

You can stretch morning or night. Once you start, it feels so good, you won't want to miss a single routine. If you do skip a day, your body will remind you. So start thinking about what time of day works best for you.

And as you'll see in Appendix B, I give you stretching routines broken down by time. If you've got 10 minutes, you can stretch. If you have 30 minutes to devote to stretching, all the better! You'll find routines for these and other amounts of time so you can work stretching into your personal   schedule.

## Stretch to Heal

Stretching is not a substitute for medical treatment when joints, muscles, or other body parts are severely injured. But it is always a part of physical therapy after treatment ends and healing begins. And it can improve the uncomfortable symptoms of a variety of ailments. So if you're suffering from a chronic illness, don't be shy about asking your doctor or physical therapist about how stretching can help you regain your health.

A regular stretching program promotes health even in an unhealthy body by improving, reversing, or eliminating all of these:

- Back and neck pain
- Arthritis
- Digestive problems
- Insomnia
- Fatigue
- Weakened immune system

## Stretching Keeps You Aligned and in Balance

Most health-care professionals agree that when your spine is in proper alignment, your whole body functions more efficiently. Stretching is, therefore, integral to correct body function, as it kicks off a series of healthful benefits in your body. Stretching ...

- Elongates and aligns your spinal column, enabling energy to flow freely.
- Helps your body better rejuvenate tissues.
- Helps relieve chronic tension.
- Helps realign muscle fibers, nerves, and fascia.

In short, stretching helps prevent painful, illnesses-causing symptoms. Like a form of massage therapy, stretching helps you relax and rest to heal injuries and make a full recovery.

The demands of work and play on specific body parts may promote *structural misalignment*. For instance, one hand moves your computer's mouse. Tennis makes use of one arm. Football relies heavily on the legs. Hips twist in one direction during a golf swing. You write with one hand. In these situations, imbalances occur as we consciously employ one or more body parts. But just as often, imbalances occur from unconscious tendencies to favor one side of the body or limb abnormally during regular daily activities.

### Flexicon

**Structural misalignment** is when the body's natural posture is altered due to gravity, the stress of daily activities, or physical injuries.

Stretching is a useful remedy for correcting structural misalignments. Each part of your body performs separate asymmetrical and symmetrical movements in a full range of motion. No other exercise gives your entire body the same even treatment like stretching.

Always stretch your body evenly by performing the same stretch on both sides of your body. For example, when you stretch your right leg, be sure you stretch your left leg, too. Stretch your left arm and then your right. One side and then the other.

# Anyone Can Stretch

Perhaps you want to start stretching because you've always yearned to touch your toes. It's not to late to start, no matter how young or old you are.

Are you an athlete who needs to make stretching part of your training regimen so you can stay at the top of your game? You've come to the right place. In Chapter 9, I give specific stretches for several sports, including the following:

◆ Walking
◆ Running
◆ Hiking
◆ Cycling
◆ Swimming
◆ Golf
◆ Tennis

### S-t-r-e-t-c-h It Out

If your sport isn't covered in this list, I also offer some sport stretching basics so you can create your own sport-specific stretching routine.

Whatever your reason, stretching is adjustable to your needs, flexibility, time, age, etc. So release any thoughts about your lack of stretchability. Flexibility is *not* a requirement. Age and fitness level do not matter. Just make stretching work for *you*—I'll show you how in the following pages—and then reap the rewards.

# A Note of Caution Before You Start

Although stretching is a safe, gentle form of exercise, it's smart to always consult your doctor before you begin a stretching program (or any exercise program) if you have a medical condition or if you are pregnant. *Contraidications* require specific precautions that are covered in the stretch descriptions in later chapters.

**Flexicon** _____

A **contraindication** is a condition that prohibits you from engaging in a particular stretch.

Above all, always listen to your body. You know it and how it moves better than anyone else. If a stretch doesn't feel right, back off.

## The Least You Need to Know

- ◆ Stretching is the activity of contracting and releasing muscles to lengthen, strengthen, and lubricate them.

- ◆ You help sustain, nourish, and relax your body and at the same time increase vitality when you stretch.

- ◆ Stretching releases stress by reducing physical, mental, and emotional tensions as you relax and unwind.

- ◆ Heal yourself as you stretch by realigning your spinal column and addressing structural misalignments.

- ◆ You don't have to be flexible to stretch.

# In This Chapter

- Understanding elasticity and movement
- Essential steps to launching your stretching program
- Exploring key stretching styles
- Breathing fundamentals
- Tips on tuning in
- Limbering up

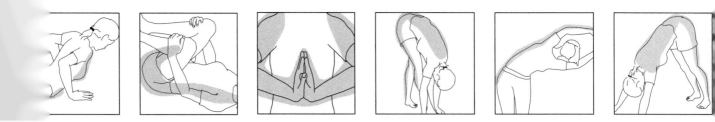

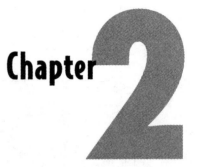

# Chapter 2

# Stretching Basics

Have you ever wanted to start something new but didn't know where to begin? If you're ready to see how you can fit stretching into your life but you're not what to do first, you've turned to the right chapter. In these pages, you learn the necessary steps to initiate your stretching routine, to ensure you're on your way to a bendable body.

Here you discover the major methods commonly used today to lengthen your muscles. You'll master vital breathing techniques to maximize your stretch and release stress. I give you tips on focusing your attention on what you're doing, to save time and energy and to prevent injuries. Finally, you can apply what you've learned and get underway as you practice important warm-ups.

## Anatomy of Elasticity

Your amazing body is structured by a skeleton with 206 bones that make up 20 percent of your total weight. Actually, you were originally born with 270 bones. You don't remember losing any, you say? That's because they're still in your body, but they're fused together. For example, your sacrum, a triangular bone at the base of your spine, consisted of six separate bones at your birth but formed a single, solid structure as you grew.

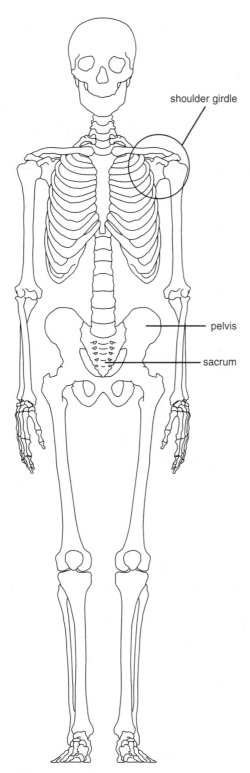

shoulder girdle

pelvis

sacrum

**Your skeleton is your body's frame, its structure.**

Your skeleton gives your body both structure and mobility. Bones protect internal organs and facilitate movement. *Ligaments*, tendons, muscles, *fascia*, cartilage, and other organs support your bones.

**Flexicon**

**Ligaments** are short bands of tough connective tissue that connect bones to other bones to form a joint. **Fascia** is specialized connective tissue surrounding muscles, bones, and joints. Fascia provides your body support, protection, and structure.

Your spine is the axis of your skeleton, linking various physiological systems to your brain—in effect, connecting your mind and body. The spine supports your trunk, which houses vital organs and acts as the base for your legs and arms. At the lower end of your trunk is your pelvis, and at the upper end is your shoulder girdle, both connected by a vertebral column crowned on the top by your head.

Have you ever observed how a baby can curl up nose to toes? That's because a baby's spine is flexible and soft. Once we learn to walk, however, our backs tighten and our spines eventually become heavy and stiff as adults. Everyday movements don't improve this condition, which is why many people suffer from back pain. But by moving the soft tissue around your spine to restore its elasticity, you can strengthen the muscles that support your spine and keep it strong and supple.

## Your Stretching Ritual

You can help maintain your flexibility with a regular stretching routine. Plan to stretch at least three times a week or as often as you exercise. Incorporate a cool-down stretch as well, when your muscles are warm and more receptive. Consistency is the key to success!

You can treat your stretching routine as seriously as you would a ritual or as casually as if by happenstance. It's your own choice. However you decide, do practice in loose, comfortable clothing and on an empty stomach, with bare feet and long hair tied back to reduce distraction. The serious stretcher should choose a quiet place, free from commotion, with enough room to stand, sit, and lie on a comfortable nonskid surface. If you choose to stretch at the gym or in your office, just grab this guide and go.

Have you determined the right time of day to start your routine? Early risers might prefer stretching after a warm shower has loosened up sleepy muscles or after 5 to 10 minutes of walking or running.

**Flex Alert!** _____

Morning stretchers should practice the warm-ups later in this chapter to prevent strains or injuries.

Not a morning person? Stretching is a great way to make the transition from work to evening relaxation. And because your muscles are already loosened up from the day's activities, you won't need as much of a warm-up.

# Mindful Stretching

Although our attention is usually directed away from our bodies, stretching draws your awareness inward. Observe how your body is responding. Which body parts are stiff or flexible, strong or weak? Do you feel ill or notice any imbalances?

As an opportunity to stop and take a look at yourself, stretching may alert you to unknown problems by uncovering hidden areas of stress, tightness, or pain. In this manner, you can make

careful, intelligent decisions about how to proceed. The more you stretch, the more you'll fine-tune your routine and know what feels right for you. Consequently, you'll make choices that promote health.

So turn off the TV and go stretch. It might be your best insurance yet!

**A Stretch in Time ...** _____

While waiting in line at the bank or supermarket, keep your feet parallel, even with your hips, and in contact with the ground. Pull in your chin, place your weight on your heels, and practice good posture.

# Dynamic and Static Stretching

You'll find two kinds of stretching in this book, *dynamic stretching* and *static stretching*.

**Flexicon** _____

**Dynamic stretching** is when you move your body in and out of the stretch, allowing your body to adjust to the stretch before you hold it. **Static stretching** is when you place your body in a stretch and hold the stretch for a number of breaths.

Dynamic stretching warms up your body, "wakes up" your muscles, and loosens your joints before you exercise or practice stronger stretches. If you're new to stretching, practice dynamic stretches for a few months to let your body gradually adjust before holding a static stretch. Dynamically stretching the sides of your body, you begin standing straight and then sway your hips one direction and your torso the other, making a half-moon shape. Moving your body from standing tall to leaning to one side and then back to standing straight provides your body with a dynamic side stretch.

Static stretches keep your body still. They are always performed after warming up or practicing dynamic stretches. For the best results, hold each static stretch for at least 30 seconds or the time required to take four long, deep breaths. Your muscles will relax and elongate when you're patient and focused on your body. After you've practiced the dynamic side stretch, holding your body in the half-moon shape, side stretch position four breaths creates a static stretch.

> **Flex Alert!** _____
>
> Never force, strain, or bounce when you stretch. Bouncing can cause small tears in your muscles, which leave scar tissue when the muscle heals. Move your body slowly and evenly during a dynamic stretch, and relax into a static stretch.

# PNF Stretching

You probably never think about how you can automatically tell where your body parts are without even having to look at them. You can reach down and scratch an itch on your knee without first having to visually locate it with your eyes, for example. This ability is called *proprioception*, which, in layman's terms, means your "sense of self." Handily, your body is equipped with proprioceptors, or sensors that provide you with this self-knowledge, such as the angle of a joint or the tension and length of a muscle as you stretch.

> **Flexicon** _____
>
> **Proprioception** is your natural sense of the position of the parts of your body in relation to each other.

Proprioceptive neuromuscular facilitation (PNF) is a stretching technique based on this sense of self, and it may help you feel your stretches more deeply. Here's how it works:

1. Either with a partner or on your own, place your body in a static stretch such as the Hamstring Stretch with Hands (Chapter 4); One Leg Up, One Leg Down (Chapters 8 and 9); or the Standing Quadriceps Stretch (Chapters 4 and 9). (Wait to come back and try this exercise after you've made it that far in the book, if you prefer.)

2. Create resistance in the stretch for 10 seconds (for example, press your leg into your hands and your hands into your leg).

3. Relax the press for 10 seconds.

4. Repeat this process two more times.

5. Stretch again, holding the final stretch for 30 seconds.

The PNF technique is a way of enhancing your stretch by pressing one part of your body against another to create a feeling of resistance—for example, pressing your hand on top of your thigh at the same time as you press your thigh into your hand. You apply this technique during a specific stretch to move your body deeper into the stretch. You would not practice the PNF technique during a dynamic stretch; it's used only while you are holding a stretch.

# Breathing Into Your Stretch

Your body has an instinctive ability and hunger to breathe deeply. Breathing fully while you're stretching calms your mind, gives you more energy, and establishes a central focus for your routine.

Observe your breath for a few moments before you start, for a perfect transition between regular activity and your stretching program.

1. Breathe with your mouth closed, through your nostrils, keeping both relaxed and passive.
2. Inhale into your upper chest, first expanding your rib cage and then your abdomen.
3. On your exhale, contract your abdominal muscles, moving your navel toward your spine.
4. Breathe in and out in a smooth and uniform flow. (Your inhale and exhale should be of equal lengths.)

You may find a natural urge to hold your breath as you move and stretch. If so, slow down the speed of your movements. Avoid jerky, irregular motions to keep your breath fluid. Notice a natural pause at the end of your inhale and exhale. If your breath is labored or your body becomes fatigued, shaky, or excessively sweaty, take a break. Use your breath as your guide.

**S-t-r-e-t-c-h It Out**

Practice breathing into your chest and exhaling from your tummy by standing and placing one hand on your chest and the other on your tummy. Inhale into your upper hand, and exhale from your lower hand.

Breathing is the most available resource you have for creating and sustaining your vital energy, and stretching is a natural way to develop your breathing. Bending backward, your chest expands and your breath naturally flows in. Bending forward, you fold your body, expelling your breath. Twists compress the right and left sides of the chest, shifting the flow of breath from one lung to the other.

Whether you can breathe deeply depends upon the nature of the stretch, so don't struggle to breathe deeply on each and every stretch.

All dynamic stretches in this book include specific instructions about when to inhale and exhale. They are always performed in coordination with the breath. This synchronization, or *envelope breathing*, makes your movements smooth and graceful.

**Flexicon**

**Envelope breathing** means to "envelop" your movements with breath. Start to breathe before you move, and end your movement with breath to spare. The flow of your breath naturally inspires and initiates the movement.

Even in static stretches, subtle movement occurs as your inhale expands your body and your exhale contracts it. Your breath ratio in a static stretch is the same as in a dynamic stretch: breathe just as deeply when you are holding a stretch as when you are stretching dynamically.

# Listening to Your Body

Stretching shouldn't be a struggle. A truly safe stretch is gentle and soothing. If you do feel resistance, mild discomfort, or a warm sensation in your muscles, relax, breathe, and hold your stretch until you feel a slight pull but no pain—this is your *edge*.

**Flexicon**

Your **edge** is a place of neither too much nor too little stretch. This place marks the healthy limit of your body's flexibility, and the place where your mind is naturally focused.

As you hold the stretch, you'll gradually feel less tension in your muscles, to the point that you can increase the stretch again until you feel the same slight pull. Continue this rhythm until you can no longer increase your stretch without pain or discomfort.

As you start your stretching program, at times you might experience both discomfort and pain. Learning to discriminate between these two sensations is crucial for safe stretching. *Discomfort* usually occurs when your body's stiffness resists the new movements of your stretching routine. You'll feel a pulling sensation, which is normal. When you do encounter discomfort, exhale deeply to relax your muscles and connective tissue.

**Flex Alert!** _____

Avoid locking your joints in place during stretches. Keep your joints and muscles relaxed to start, and gradually extend your arms and legs, remembering always to keep a slight bend in your elbows and knees while you stretch. It's essential not to push beyond your body's natural elasticity.

*Pain,* however, is an obvious warning sign that you have exceeded healthy limits and are risking injury. If you feel pain as you stretch, you've gone past your body's natural restrictions. Pain may appear as a sudden, sharp, or shooting sensation, or occur after an injury as a throb or ache. The knees, back, and neck are three common sites of pain caused by sports, unrelieved sitting, and the sedentary nature of work. Steer clear of any stretch that places stress or pressure on the affected body part, especially right after you feel pain.

If your shoulders are stressed, try keeping your arms raised over your head. If your knees are injured, pad them with a folded blanket. As pain diminishes, choose stretches that gently move the affected part of your body.

**S-t-r-e-t-c-h It Out** _____

Is your natural tendency to stretch beyond your body's healthy flexibility limit or short of your "edge"? The optimum stretch stops at the relaxed side of your edge, the place where your breath flows smoothly and you feel a sense of accomplishment. Watch how your edge changes as you progress.

# Warming Up

Always stretch only after you've warmed up your body, to prevent injury and increase your range of motion. Warm-ups raise your pulse rate and core body temperature, and encourage deeper breathing. Cold, tight muscles and connective tissue loosen, and joints become lubricated with *synovial fluid.* Coordination and circulation improve as your muscles adjust to the idea of expanding and contracting. You'll also awaken your mind and nervous system, leading to increased awareness and greater body sensitivity.

**Flexicon** _____

**Synovial fluid** is a thin, stringy liquid found in joint cavities that reduces friction between cartilage and other tissues. Synovial fluid lubricates and cushions joints during movement.

Taking the time to warm up honors your body's need to move gradually into movement and deeper stretching. Keep it simple. Practice the following dynamic stretches as a precursor to holding a static stretch. Five to ten minutes of easy walking or jogging, or practicing these warm-ups ensures you'll be stretching free of injury for many years to come.

## Morning Stretch

Are you an early stretcher? Then this warm-up's for you. You can even practice it before you get out of bed, to get a jump-start on your program.

1. Before you begin, either while lying down or standing up with your feet together, imagine you are standing on the floor, feet and heels anchored. Be sure you have enough room over your head to sweep your arms back without hitting the wall.
2. Inhale deeply as your arms move up toward the ceiling and over your head, move slowly to feel your ribs and chest expand.
3. With your arms overhead, pause for a moment and feel the fullness of your breath.
4. Feel the entire back of your body as you exhale, returning your arms to your sides.
5. As you exhale reach deeply through your heels to intensify the stretch.

The following warm-up is wonderful for those times when you're stuck in bed or feeling under the weather.

1. Lie on your back, arms at your sides, your feet flexed and even with your hips. Close your eyes for a moment, take a deep breath, and relax your whole body as you exhale. Notice the entire back of your body.

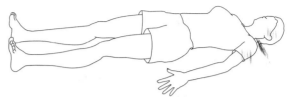

To begin the Morning Stretch, lie supine (on your back) with your arms at your sides.

2. S-t-r-e-t-c-h your arms up toward the ceiling, over your head, and toward the floor behind you, inhaling as you move. Envelop your movements with your breath. Pause.

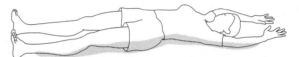

Stretch your arms over your head toward the floor.

3. Exhale. Extend your arms toward the ceiling and back down to your sides. Pause.
4. Repeat these movements three more times.

**S-t-r-e-t-c-h It Out**

The shaded part of each figure, as in the preceding figure, shows which area of the body is stretched.

## Bicycling

Bicycling your legs is a playful way to warm up your body without placing any strain on your back. Rotating the large bones and muscles of your legs quickly raises your heart rate and body temperature, strengthens your abdominal muscles, and lubricates your hip and knee joints. Rotate your legs evenly and smoothly, as if you were actually riding a bicycle.

1. Lie on your back, with your arms beside your body for stability. Draw your knees toward your chest as you exhale.

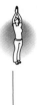

**Flex Alert!** _____

Sore back? Support it by placing your hands under your lower back, palms down, elbows slightly bent out to the sides of your torso.

2. Rotate your legs forward, making full circles as if you were riding a bicycle. Keep breathing as you move. Start with 30 cycles, eventually working your way up to 50.

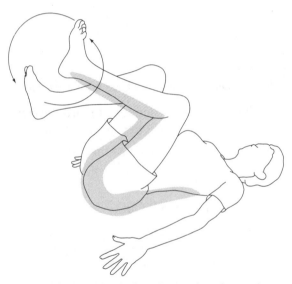

**Lying on your back, bicycle your legs forward.**

3. Now reverse the direction, rotating your legs backward, cycling in the same manner as in step 2. Continue to breathe as you move. The reverse direction might seem awkward, so concentrate on moving as smoothly as you can. Begin with 30 circles and then progress slowly to 50.

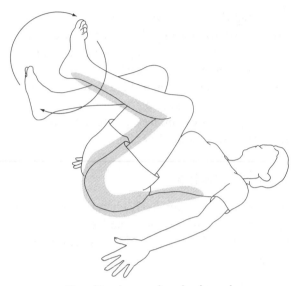

**Now bicycle your legs backward.**

Observe yourself closely as you bicycle backward. Can you move as smoothly as in the forward rotation? Are you remembering to breathe?

4. Hold your knees and rest for a moment.

## Gentle Twist

Wake up your spine and massage your internal organs with this gentle warm-up—but do proceed with caution if your back is injured. You may gradually deepen the twist with each repetition, but novices should keep their knees directly above their hips. Experienced stretchers may place their knees closer to their chests.

Keep your shoulders and neck relaxed, and practice a long exhale with a little pause at the end as you hold the twist.

1. Lie on your back, with your arms away from your body to form a T, palms up. Draw your knees toward your chest as you exhale.

4. Repeat steps 2 and 3 two more times, and hold the twist on each side for four breaths.

5. Finish on your back, holding your knees while you rest for a few breaths.

### S-t-r-e-t-c-h It Out

Studies show that holding a stretch for 30 seconds is an effective component of conditioning plans that improve range of motion. Four long breaths should ensure that you're sufficiently holding your stretches. Everyone breathes at a different rate, so time your breathing and adjust the number of breaths accordingly.

## Spinal Roll

Practicing this warm-up every day keeps your spine supple. Start slowly, lifting your hips only until you feel a nice stretch up the front of your thighs and across your upper back. With each repetition, you may raise your hips higher, but not if you feel tightness in your lower back. Keep your head straight at all times, and relax your shoulders and neck as much as possible. Try to feel each vertebra in your upper back, the middle of your back, and, finally, your lower back as you unwind your spine down to the floor.

1. Lie on your back, your feet close to your buttocks and even with your hips. Bring your arms to your sides, palms down. Exhale fully.

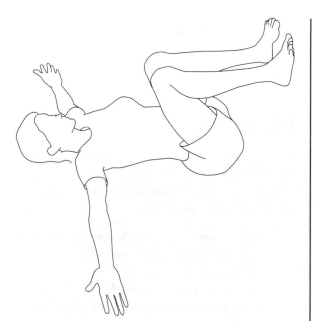

To begin the Gentle Twist, lie on your back, your arms away from your body like a T, palms up, knees toward your chest.

2. Inhale and slowly move both knees to one side of your body as you exhale. Pause for a moment as you breathe in.

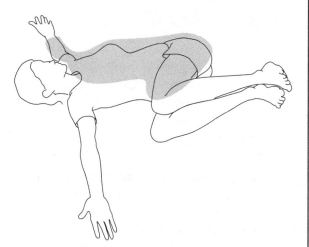

Slowly move your knees to the right as you exhale.

3. Lift your knees back to the starting position as you exhale. Then repeat the twist, this time lowering your knees to the opposite side.

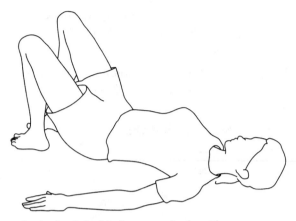

**Begin the Spinal Roll on your back, with your arms at your sides and your feet hip-width apart on the floor.**

2. Inhale as you press into your feet, lifting your hips, simultaneously lifting your arms first toward the ceiling and then back over your head toward the floor, resting them behind you.

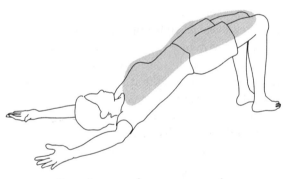

**Press into your feet as you stretch.**

3. Slowly lower your spine and, at the same time, return your arms to their starting position.
4. Repeat these movements three more times using your envelope breathing.
5. Draw your knees to your chest as you exhale, and hold your knees and rest.

**Flex Alert!** _____

Skip the spinal roll warm-up if your back is injured.

## Hamstring Stretch

The two sequential movements that make up the Hamstring Stretch wake up your hips, strengthen your abdominals, and stretch your lower back and hamstrings.

1. Lie on your back, your knees bent, with your feet on the floor, even with and a comfortable distance away from your hips. Rest your arms beside your body. Draw your knees toward your chest as you exhale.

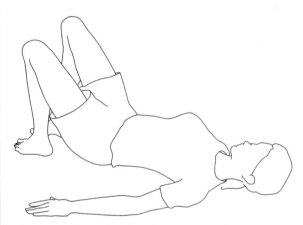

**Begin the Hamstring Stretch on your back, your arms at your sides, your feet hip-width apart on the floor.**

2. Lift your feet toward the ceiling as you inhale deeply, straightening your legs and raising your arms back over your head toward the floor behind you. You can keep a bend in your knees if your hamstrings are tight. Keep your lower back flat on the floor.

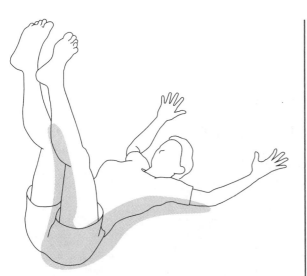

**Stretch out your hamstrings while remembering to breathe.**

3. Bend your knees toward your chest, hands on your knees, curling up like a ball as you exhale. Keep your head on the floor.

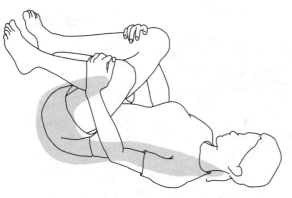

**Use your hands on your knees to deepen the stretch.**

4. Repeat steps 2 and 3 three more times, moving while you breathe, and then hold your knees and rest.

## The Least You Need to Know

◆ Stretch at least three times a week or as often as you exercise to receive the maximum benefits of stretching.

◆ Stretching dynamically acts as a warm-up, allowing your body to adjust to holding a stretch.

◆ Breathe deeply into your upper chest and flatten your tummy as you exhale. Envelop your movements with breath.

◆ Learn the difference between pain and discomfort as you stretch. Practice stretching at the comfortable side of your edge.

◆ Always practice warm-ups to remain injury-free.

# In This Part

3  Opening the Top of Your Body

4  Hips, Legs, Thighs, and Feet—Your Base

5  Stretching Your Whole Body

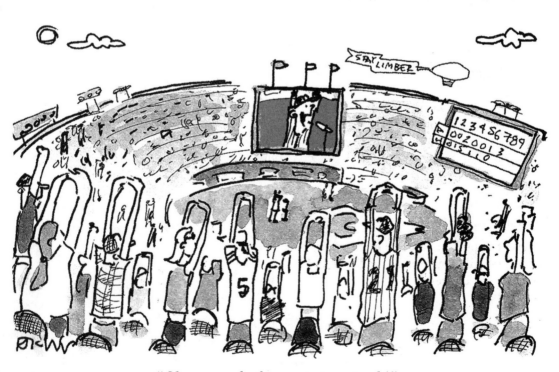

*"Okay, everybody, now s-t-r-e-t-c-h!"*

# Stretching from Head to Toe

Part 2 teaches you how to stretch, starting at the top of your body, and moving downward to your feet and ending with whole body routines. Breathe freely as you practice stretches that expand your chest and lungs, and release tension from your waist to your crown. These stretches help improve your posture with specific routines guaranteed to unlock your jaw, soothe your eyes, untie knots in your neck and shoulders, loosen wrist joints, and relax your hands. Then, you'll stretch from hips to heels. No time for a comprehensive program? Also included are six essential ways to stretch your body.

# In This Chapter

◆ Release tension from waist to crown

◆ Unlock your jaw and soothe your eyes

◆ Untie knots in your neck and shoulders, loosen your wrist joints, and stretch your hands

◆ Breathe easier with stretches that expand your chest and lungs

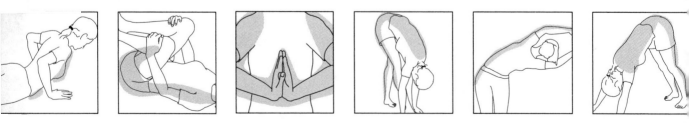

# Chapter 3

# Opening the Top of Your Body

You learned the basics of stretching in Chapter 2; now it's time to work your way, systematically, throughout the body, starting from the top. Don't worry if you're just beginning, are elderly, or are dealing with an illness: these moves are perfect for everyone, especially those who have been advised to avoid vigorous physical exercise. Simple, gentle, and comfortable, stretching the top of your body relaxes tense muscles caused by writing, typing, driving, and doing office work.

Have you ever had to adjust your car's rear view mirror before you drive home from work? That's because you're actually shorter than you were at the beginning of the day. Why? Blame it on the earth's gravity, which gradually compresses your spine. So imagine gravity's effect over the course of your lifetime. Normal curvatures of your spine don't remain intact as you age. Your shoulders become more rounded and stooped, your head lifts to look forward, and your abdomen bulges. These changes caused by gravity are worsened by a decline in your muscle strength.

Top-of-the body stretches can prevent or offset the tendency of spinal curvatures to slump or deform with age. They can also strengthen and stretch your eye muscles; release tension in your jaw, wrists, and hands; and prevent your upper back and shoulders from rounding, collapsing your chest.

# The Head Leads the Way

Your head weighs about 10 pounds—none of which you'll ever want to lose. Housing your brain and covered with the muscles of your face and scalp, your head contains the sensory organs that guide you through the world. Your face—with its eyes, ears, nose, and mouth—is the central locus of four senses: seeing, hearing, smelling, and tasting. The muscles of your face that let you smile, frown, raise your eyebrows, or wrinkle your forehead are as important expressions as the sounds and words you create using your tongue and teeth, which, in conjunction with your jaw, also allow you to chew and ingest your food. Indeed, the interconnected functions of each component of your head are what make you "you," what give you your primary experience and identity. So why would you want to overlook stretching them for good health?

Eye stretches strengthen and stretch the muscles that perform the important tasks of looking, watching, and observing. They re-establish balance and develop coordination in the muscles that surround your eyes, as well as improve your ability to focus on an object.

**Flex Alert!** _____

If you suffer from any major eye diseases or disorders, consult an eye specialist before performing eye stretches.

All stretches start in a seated position with your eyeglasses removed. Before you begin, you may splash cold water onto your eyes to stimulate their blood supply. Keep your facial muscles, eyebrows, and eyelids relaxed as you stretch. After each stretch, close and rest your eyes for four deep breaths. You may also place your palms over your eyes to soothe them.

Perform eye stretches with patience and determination, once in the morning and once in the evening. Don't expect instant results; it takes time and practice before you see progress. But you will.

## Eagle Eye Stretch

Before you begin, give your eyes a break. Sit quietly and rub your hands together briskly to create heat in your palms. Close your eyes and gently cover them with your warm palms. Feel your eye muscles softening as they bathe in soothing darkness. Consciously release the muscles that surround your eyes, and breathe deeply. Once your eyes have absorbed the heat, lower your hands, keeping your eyes closed. Repeat this relaxing sequence twice before you begin stretching. As you perform this routine, inhale as your arm ascends and exhale as it descends.

1. Sit in a comfortable position, your spine straight. Rest your left hand on your left thigh. Stretch your right arm in front of you, elbow straight, hand in a fist, right thumb pointing up toward the sky.

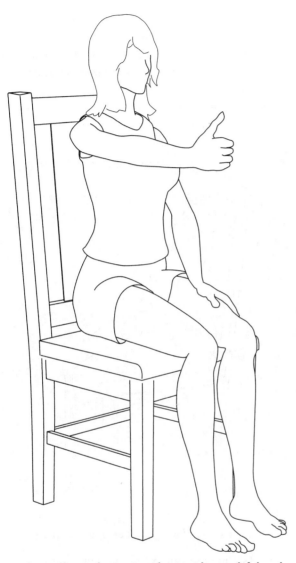

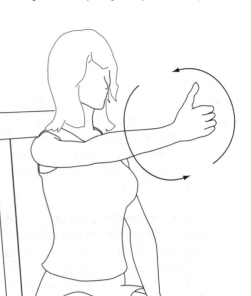

**To begin the Eagle Eye Stretch, sit with your left hand on your left thigh, and raise your right arm forward, fisted hand, thumb up.**

2. Raise your right arm toward the ceiling, to the left, down toward your legs, and then to your right, making a large circle, ending in the starting position. Focus your eyes on your thumb while your head remains still, facing forward.

**Circle your right arm to the left, watching it with your eyes without moving your head.**

3. Repeat step 2 five times in each direction.
4. Repeat steps 2 and 3 with your left thumb.
5. Finish by closing and resting your eyes, or by warming your palms by rubbing them together and placing them over your closed eyes.

## Eye Push-Ups

Before you begin Eye Push-Ups, relax your eyes as you did for the Eagle Eye Stretch. In this stretch, you'll bring your thumb to the tip of your nose, hold it there as you take a full breath, and exhale as you move it away. When finished, be sure to rest your eyes by closing them or repeating the relaxation sequence from the beginning.

1. Sit in a comfortable position, your spine straight. Rest your left hand on your left thigh. Stretch your right arm in front of you at shoulder level. Your elbow should be straight and your hand rolled into a fist, with your thumb pointing upward.

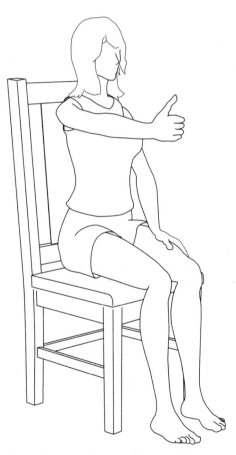

To begin Eye Push-Ups, sit with your left hand on your left thigh, and raise your right arm forward, fisted hand, thumb up.

2. Gaze at your thumb as you bend your arm to bring your thumb to your nose. Take a full breath as you hold your thumb at the tip of your nose, still gazing at your thumb.

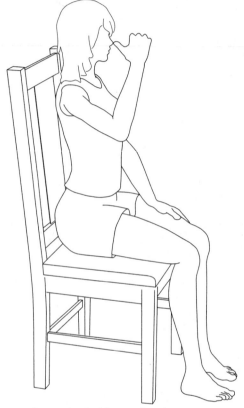

Breathe as you hold your thumb to your nose.

3. As you continue watching your thumb, slowly straighten your arm back to the starting position.

4. Repeat this sequence four more times and then close and rest your eyes for a few moments before repeating on the left side.

 **A Stretch in Time ...**

Pairing a stretch with an activity you perform every day is a good way to work stretching into your day without stress. Try practicing Eye Push-Ups before you brush your teeth.

## Jolly Jaws

Jaw stretches release tension in your jaw, a common body part where many people hold stress. Have you ever awakened with a stiff or sore jaw? That's probably caused by unconsciously clenching your teeth while you sleep. During the day, chewing gum may exacerbate the pain and tension.

This simple stretch works wonders for releasing a tense jaw. Practice Jolly Jaws morning and night, focusing your attention on your proper sitting posture and stretching sensations. When you've completed this stretch, sit for a few moments and enjoy the aftermath.

1. Sit in a cross-legged position on the floor or in a comfortable chair, keeping your spine and legs straight and your feet on the floor directly below your knees. Bend your elbows and rest your hands on your thighs.

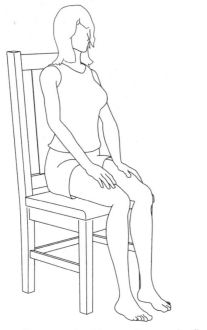

To begin Jolly Jaws, sit with your feet on the floor below your knees, with your hands resting on your thighs.

2. Draw in a deep breath as you raise your shoulders toward your ears. Pause, hold your breath for a moment, and drop your shoulders away from your ears. Relax.

3. Hold your mouth open as wide as possible for 10 seconds. Close your mouth and repeat three to five times. You may close your eyes and rest them as you practice if you want.

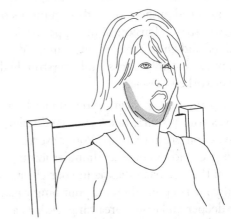

To really stretch your jaw, open your mouth w-i-d-e and hold it for 10 seconds.

# Upper Back, Shoulders, and Chest

Many factors can cause chronic upper-body tension and changes to your posture: aging, gravity, anxiety, driving, typing, carrying heavy weight, slouching, shrugging—the list goes on. Before you know it, you may find yourself habitually standing with the tops of your shoulders rolled in or your head pushed forward—symptoms of unrelieved stress. Tension of the upper back, shoulders, and chest can also result in headaches, muscular imbalances, and overstretched and overworked muscles.

Taking the time to stretch your upper body improves your posture, helps you stand taller, and gives you greater vitality. You preserve the range of motion in your shoulder joints, lengthen the *intercostal muscles* in your chest, expand your rib cage, increase your lung capacity for deeper and easier breathing, and, as a result, boost your energy level. But before you begin these routines, consult your physician if you have pain, weakness, or numbness in your neck, arms, shoulders, upper back, hands, or fingers.

**Flexicon** _____

**Intercostal muscles** are several groups of muscles that run between the ribs and help form and move the chest wall.

## Sun and Earth

Sun and Earth is a great routine for warming up your back and shoulders as you expand your chest. Practice this dynamic sequence to prepare your body for the rest of the stretches in this chapter, and then again after your stretches as a cool-down.

Keep your body comfortable, balanced, and stable as you move. If you feel pain, consider it a warning and stop. Remember to use envelope breathing evenly as you go.

1. On a mat or blanket, sit on your heels, rest your hands on your thighs, and notice where you feel a stretch.

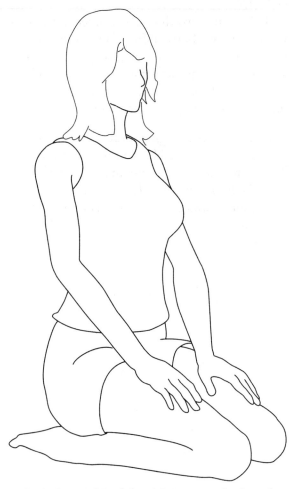

**Begin Sun and Earth by sitting on your heels and resting your hands on your thighs. Where do you feel the stretch?**

**S-t-r-e-t-c-h It Out** _____

Use an extra folded blanket to kneel on when practicing Sun and Earth. Your knees will thank you.

2. Sweep your arms wide, making a big circle like the sun, and inhale as you lift your hips off your heels. Stretch your arms over your head and bring your palms together. You may keep your arms shoulder-width apart if your shoulders are tight.

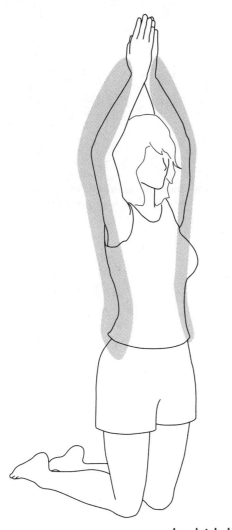

**As you sweep your arms up over your head, inhale and raise to a standing position on your knees.**

3. As you exhale, bend forward, sweeping your arms wide until the backs of your hands land on your lower back, palms turned upward.

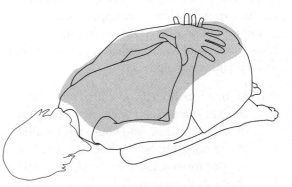

**On the exhale, fold forward over your knees and rest the backs of your hands on your lower back, your palms turned upward.**

4. As you inhale, lift your hips up off your heels and continue moving through steps 2 and 3 four more times.

6. To finish, sit on your heels and rest with your hands on your thighs.

**S-t-r-e-t-c-h It Out** _____

Don't be alarmed if you experience cramps in your feet when practicing Sun and Earth. Once your feet become accustomed to the idea of stretching, the cramps should subside. If not, you may always consult your health-care provider. To ease a cramping foot, stop and massage your foot. Massaging your feet every morning with sesame oil and taking hot baths helps relieve cramps and soreness, too. See Chapter 4 for more on care for your feet.

# Pretzel

The name of this stretch might sound intimidating, but don't be concerned—you won't be contorting your body in the shape of a pretzel. Use this routine when your upper back is sore or tight, but don't overdo it, as this stretch keeps your shoulders rounded. And remember to keep your chest open.

1. Sit in a sturdy chair on a firm seat with a straight spine. Keep your jaw loose, your shoulders relaxed, and your chin parallel to the floor. Straighten both arms in front of your torso at shoulder level, your palms skyward. Bend your right elbow, and place it in the crease of your left elbow.

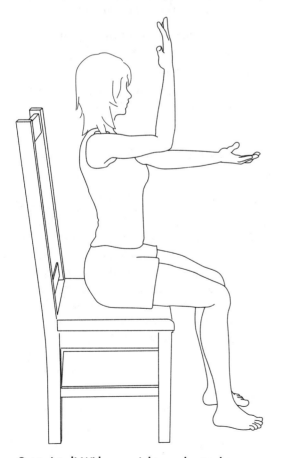

Get twisted! With your right arm bent, place your right elbow in the crease of your left arm.

2. Entwine your arms until you can place the fingers of your left hand on your right palm. If you can't touch your fingers to your palm, bring them to your wrist or forearm in a loose wrap.

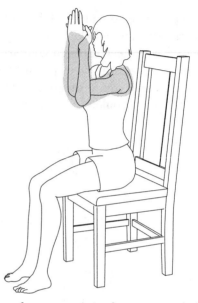

With your forearms entwined, you can probably see where this stretch gets its name.

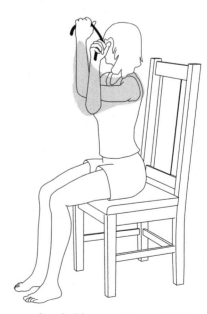

If you need to, hold a strap in your left hand and grasp it with your right hand.

3. Move your elbows up or down slowly until you find your edge, and hold the stretch for four deep breaths, sitting steady. Each time you inhale, imagine your upper back expanding. Picture your upper-back muscles becoming soft and pliable as you exhale. You may close your eyes to notice where you feel the stretch in your body.

4. Release your arms, let your hands rest on your thighs, and observe the difference in how your shoulders feel.

5. Repeat steps 1 through 4, placing your left elbow in the crease of your right elbow, and once again hold your position for four breaths, noticing any variations as you stretch this side.

## Figure Eight

Return your body to its natural alignment with the Figure Eight, and your overworked back will thank you. As you hold the stretch, you may close your eyes and picture your spine lengthening from base to crown. With every inhale, inch your upper elbow higher and your lower elbow toward the floor. Hold your body calmly with a quiet breath.

1. Sit in a sturdy chair on a firm seat with a straight spine. Keep your jaw loose, shoulders relaxed, and chin parallel to the floor. Raise your right arm over your head, bend your elbow, and place your palm between your shoulder blades.

2. Sweep your left arm back behind your torso, bend your elbow, and place your left hand in the middle of your back, palm out. Hook the fingers of your right and left hands together. Use a belt, strap, sock, or tie if your fingers cannot touch.

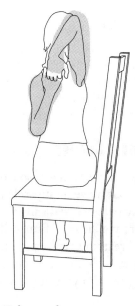

The Figure Eight stretches your arms up and back.

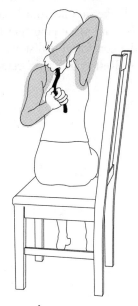

If you need to, you can use a strap.

3. Hold the stretch for four gentle breaths. Do not force or strain.

4. Let go of your fingers, allow your arms to rest with your hands on your thighs, and observe your shoulders.

5. Now practice the same stretch with your left arm up and your right arm down. Notice if one shoulder feels different.

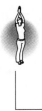

**Flex Alert!**

Keep your head aligned straight with your spine and contract your abdominal muscles as you sit, ensuring a proper posture.

## Relaxing Chest Opener

The Relaxing Chest Opener is so easy, there's nothing to do but move gently, relax, and breathe deeply (which is basically what it's all about). Be sure you lie on a firm surface and use envelope breathing. You can practice this stretch at any time, but it's particularly suitable in the evening to calm your mind after a long day.

1. Lie on your back on the floor. Use a rug, mat, or blanket to pad your back. Bend your knees and place your feet parallel with and a comfortable distance away from your hips. Rest your arms beside your body.

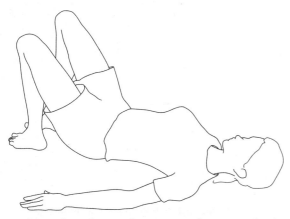

To begin the Relaxing Chest Opener, lie on your back and bend your knees, with your feet hip-width apart and parallel, and your arms at your sides.

2. Raise both arms toward the ceiling and back over your head toward the floor behind you as you inhale. Exhale your arms back down to your sides. Continue to move and breathe in this manner five more times.

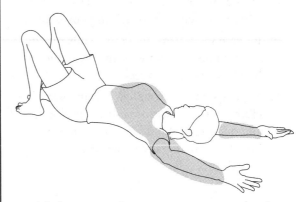

Inhale as you raise your arms over your head.

## Chest Expander

This routine helps you find your balance and proper posture as you expand your chest. Center your attention on the places you feel the stretch and on your breathing. Don't strain if you have a stiff neck. Remember your edge.

1. Stand with your feet parallel and even with your hips. Rest your arms beside your body. Tuck your chin. Inhale and then relax as you exhale, with your knees slightly bent.

2. Raise your arms out to your sides and over your head as you inhale. Interlacing your fingers at the top, press your palms up and s-t-r-e-t-c-h.

3. Bend your elbows, fingers interlaced
   and palms up, bringing your hands back
   behind your head and toward your neck as
   you exhale. Keep your chin toward your
   chest.

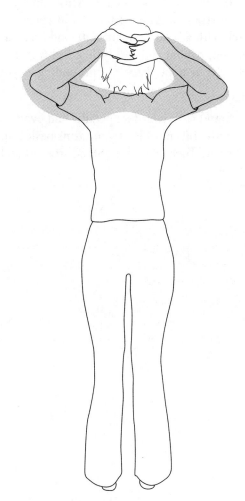

**To begin the Chest Expander, stand with your feet
parallel and hip-width apart, your arms beside your
body, and your chin tucked.**

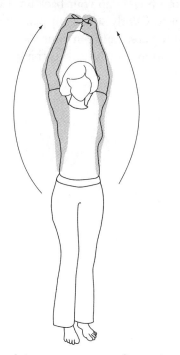

**Feel the stretch in your arms, your fingers interlaced
and palms up.**

**Bend your elbows and bring your hands behind your
head, your fingers still interlaced and palms up.**

4. Inhale and straighten your arms toward
   the ceiling with your fingers interlaced and
   palms up, as in step 2. Exhale as you lower
   your arms to the starting position.

5. Repeat steps 2 through 4 three more
   times.

# Prayer

Watch your progress as you perform this routine that stretches your fingers, palms, arms, and chest. You may start by holding your forearms or elbows, if you need to. Move slowly without strain or undue effort. Hold your stretch with a balance of strength and relaxed attention, patient and steady, like a prayer, to prevent your upper back from rounding as you age.

1. Stand with your feet parallel and even with your hips. Rest your arms beside your body. Tuck your chin. Stand straight and tall.

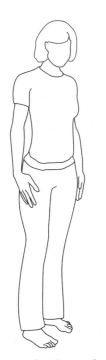

To begin Prayer, stand with your feet parallel and hip-width apart, your arms beside your body, and your chin tucked.

2. Inhaling as you move, lift your arms out to the sides and up over your head, interlocking your fingers as your palms meet. S-t-r-e-t-c-h your palms up toward the ceiling and pause.

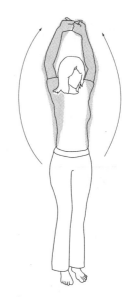

Feel the stretch in your arms, your fingers interlaced and palms up.

3. Exhale as you sweep your arms wide, making a big circle and bringing your palms together behind you at the base of your spine. If your fingers are together, you can gradually work your fingers up your back until your palms meet. Gently slide your palms up your spine to the area between your shoulder blades. Continue rhythmic breathing.

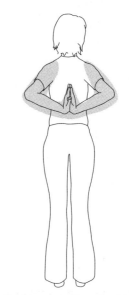

Your arms, shoulders, and hands should feel the stretch, with your palms together between your shoulder blades.

**S-t-r-e-t-c-h It Out**

If you can't bring your fingers or palms together in Prayer, hold your forearms or elbows.

4. With your chin tucked, hold the stretch for three smooth breaths. Inhale as you release your palms and stretch your arms out to the sides and up over your head, interlacing your fingers at the top. Press your palms skyward as in step 2.

5. Inhale and straighten your extended arms, palms up with your fingers interlaced, and pause at the top as in step 2. Lower your arms to your sides as you exhale. Take a moment to observe where you feel the stretch in your body.

# Wrists and Hands

Our wrists and hands are vital body parts, yet we tend to ignore them until they become injured, stiff, or sore. Our hands are our primary vehicle of touch and means of manipulating our environment, from gross motor movements such as swinging a golf club to fine motor tasks such as typing. Stretching your hands, wrists, and forearms is a welcome relief for stiff and sore joints. The following routines are excellent for those who are immobile, suffering from illness, diagnosed with arthritis, or advised not to participate in vigorous physical exercise. They're also perfect for counteracting the effects of office work, such as the tension resulting from extended periods of writing and typing.

All wrist and hand stretches start in a seated position. Engage only the muscles involved, keeping the rest of your body relaxed as you stretch. If you feel balanced and comfortable, close your eyes while you practice these stretches, to focus your attention on where

you're feeling the stretch. After each stretch, relax and notice the parts of your body you've moved. As you rest your body, you'll begin to develop an awareness of how you're feeling, which is as important as the stretches themselves.

## Finger Wrap

Do your hands ache from gripping a steering wheel or pulling on the reins of a bridle? Have you been grasping a hammer or saw? How about a rolling pin over the holiday pie-making season? If so, or if your hands are stiff and sore from other causes, try the Finger Wrap. You'll wake up each part of your hands, discover just how far you can open them, and gauge your coordination, to boot. Move slowly as you practice Finger Wrap, and if you need to rest your arms midway, please do!

1. Sit in a heavy chair and keep your spine straight. Firmly plant your feet directly under your knees. Lift both arms forward, holding them at shoulder level, with your palms down. Open your hands, reaching through your fingertips, and stretch your palms wide as you breathe in.

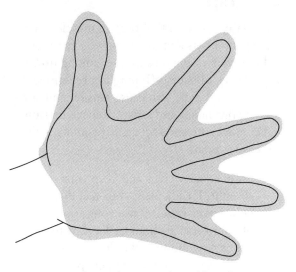

Spread your fingers wide and breathe.

2. Slowly wrap your fingers around your thumbs, pinky first, index finger last, as you exhale.

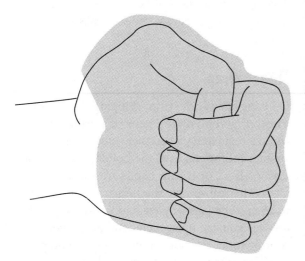

**Wrap your fingers one by one around your thumb.**

3. Repeat stretching your palms wide and wrapping your fingers around your thumbs nine more times. Mentally count each Finger Wrap as you focus on your movement and how your hands feel. Finish by resting your hands and arms.

## Wrist Waves

Wrist Waves stretch the forearm muscles that move your wrists and fingers so you can type and use your computer's mouse, among other movements, of course. Typing is a repetitive task that, over time, can cause tension and stiffness in your hands and wrists. Relieve tension and combat sore and stiff arthritic joints with this easy stretch.

1. Sit in a heavy chair and keep your spine straight. Firmly plant your feet directly under your knees. Raise your arms in front of your torso at shoulder level, with your palms down toward the floor. Bend your hands backward, your fingers pointing

upward, as if you were gesturing "stop." Inhale and then pause to feel the stretch.

2. Bend your hands forward, your fingers pointing downward as you exhale.

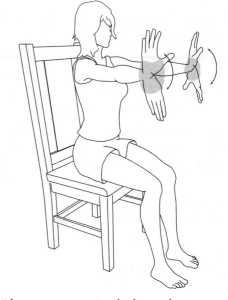

**With your arms outstretched, stretch your wrist up and down.**

3. Repeat steps 1 and 2 nine more times, breathing and counting as you move. Keep your fingers and elbows straight, your fingers together, and your palms open as if you are waving. If your arms tire, take a break and rest your hands on your thighs. Focus your mind on the movement of your wrist joint, stretch sensations, your breathing, and counting.

## Wrist Circles

Loosen painful arthritic joints; relieve tension caused by prolonged writing, typing, and driving; and increase the range of motion in your wrists by practicing Wrist Circles. As you move each wrist, you'll become aware of any differences between the two.

1. Start in a comfortable sitting posture with a straight spine. Wrap your fingers around your thumbs, making fists. Stretch your arms out at shoulder level. Rotate your fists to the right and then to the left 10 times in each direction. Watch the range of motion in each wrist, and observe any differences. Once complete, rest your hands on your thighs and take a few breaths.

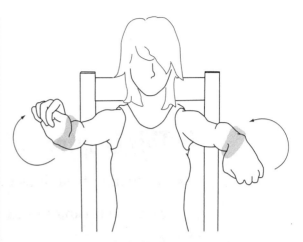

Now rotate your wrists in the opposite directions.

### A Stretch in Time ...

Master the wrist and hands stretches so you can take them with you as you move through your day. Practice these simple stretches while standing, walking, or sitting at your desk or watching television.

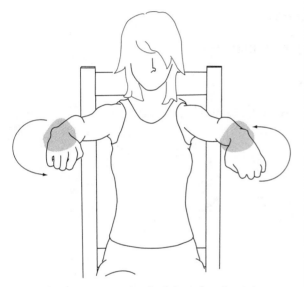

Rotate your wrists to the left and to the right.

2. Now repeat the same stretch, this time rotating your wrists in opposite directions, 10 times in each direction. Keep your mind on what you're doing as you rotate your wrists. Your elbows and arms should remain in a straight line and static throughout the movements. However, feel free to rest your arms when you need to rather than strain. Rotate your fist in as large a circle as you comfortably can. Rest your arms and hands when you're finished.

## The Least You Need to Know

- The gravity that anchors your lower body to the earth helps lengthen your spine and prevent your upper back from rounding forward as you age.

- Opening the top of your body helps you stand tall and breathe more deeply, giving you more energy and strength.

- Stretching your eye muscles and jaws assists in avoiding eyestrain and jaw pain and tension.

- As you age, the range of motion in your shoulder joints tends to diminish. Practicing upper-back, shoulder, and chest stretches may inhibit this tendency.

- Combat arthritis and keep hands and wrists pain-free by stretching these vital parts of your body.

# In This Chapter

- ◆ Stretching from hips to heels
- ◆ Stress-releasing hip stretches
- ◆ Say good-bye to your tight hamstrings
- ◆ Say hello to your quadriceps
- ◆ Protect your feet, knees, and calves with five simple stretches

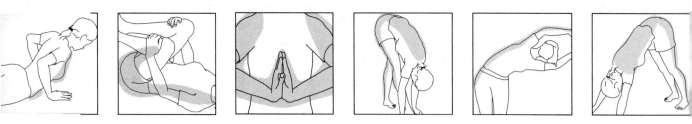

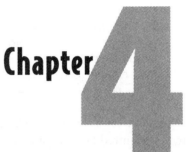

# Hips, Legs, Thighs, and Feet— Your Base

Have you ever thought of your body as a tree? When the tree's base or trunk is sturdy, the tree is stable and vital. Branches, leaves, and fruit extend upward toward the sun and sky. Like a tree, your own base should be strong and flexible to let you feel fully alive. That's why stretching your hips, thighs, and feet is so important to maintaining your entire body.

## Base Basics

Do you suffer from shortened hamstring muscles along the backs of your legs, tight *hip flexors* along the front of your thighs, or tight groin muscles and *hip rotators?* Perhaps your pelvis feels locked, forcing you to bend forward from your spine and rounding your back. Or maybe you suffer from *musculoskeletal* conditions in your lower body, such as having one hip rotated forward or higher than another.

**Flexicon**

**Hip flexors** are a set of muscles found in your pelvis that bend your hips and rotate your lower spine. **Hip rotators** are a group of six muscles that help your hips rotate either inward or outward. **Musculoskeletal** relates to your skeleton, joints, muscles, and tendons.

The source of these problems may be inherited or acquired because of injury or habitual patterns of movement, such as sitting on your wallet in your back pocket or carrying a baby on one hip. In any case, tension in your base can prevent you from fully enjoying your life and participating in activities such as riding a bike, walking, or jogging. Base stretches provide many immediate benefits: trimming and strengthening your hips, thighs, and abdominal muscles; improving circulation through your hip joints, legs, and pelvic region; stretching, toning, and lengthening your entire spinal column; and loosening spinal vertebrae, to name a few.

As you practice these routines, pay attention to the key junction where your legs connect to your spine through your pelvis. Observe how that junction feels at the front, back, outside, and inside of your legs and pelvis. Once you gain more knowledge about this area of your lower body, you can stretch the muscles you feel most need it. In so doing, you'll strengthen the muscles that support your joints and release muscle spasms or chronically contracted muscles.

**S-t-r-e-t-c-h It Out**

Always warm up and feel free to adapt any position to meet your needs. Explore what feels right by working gently, without placing any stress on your joints. Focus on long exhales as you bend forward, to facilitate the stretch and release tension. Most stretches are performed either sitting or lying on your back to relieve joint pressure.

# Hip Openers

Held together by muscles, tendons, and ligaments, your hip is the largest joint in your body. Its primary function is to support the weight of your body in static and dynamic positions. As you might guess, then, your hips sustain a great deal of wear and tear. It should be no surprise that approximately 200,000 Americans undergo total hip replacement surgery every year.

**Flex Alert!**

If you've had a hip replacement, check with your doctor before trying the hip opener stretches.

In a domino effect, tight hips can make your back tight, pull your pelvis forward, roll your thighs outward, and apply extra pressure to your knees and lower back. Rigid hip muscles can change your posture, inhibit movement, and tighten groin muscles, hip rotators, and hip flexors along the front of your thighs. These muscle imbalances may bring on a host of health problems, especially lower-back pain, which, unfortunately, can prevent you from enjoying some of your favorite activities.

You can tell whether your hips are tight by standing and looking at your feet. Do your toes naturally turn out? If so, you might need to work on opening and balancing your hip muscles. Hip opener stretches do just that and more: release stress, expand your range of motion, and lower your risk of injury.

## Diamond

Diamond is an effortless but powerful stretch for your inner thigh muscles and the nerve fibers in your groin. It helps loosen the joints in your lower body, massage the organs in your abdominal area, and strengthen your back and spine.

**Flex Alert!** _____

Skip Diamond and try the stretches in Chapter 8 if your back is sore or injured.

1. Sit on a comfortable surface with a straight spine. Bring the soles of your feet together, heels close to your groin, legs in the shape of a diamond.

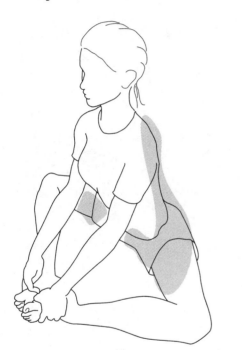

With your legs in this position, you can see where this stretch gets its name.

**S-t-r-e-t-c-h It Out** _____

If your back is stiff or sensitive, sit on the forward edge of a folded blanket to help keep your spine straight. Likewise, if you have knee pain, kneel on folded blankets for those stretches that require you to be in that position.

2. Hold your feet with your hands. If you feel your back rounding, hold your ankles or calves instead. Inhale deeply and feel your spine elongate up toward the crown of your head. Keep your spine straight, upper back flat, and chin parallel to the floor. You may move your feet away from your hips if you feel strain in your knees or groin. Don't force or strain!

3. Contract your abdominal muscles as you strongly exhale all your breath. It's okay if your body leans forward from the hips, but be sure you keep your back straight.

4. Hold this position for four long, smooth breaths, or even longer, if you want. Relax and let gravity do the work. Notice where you feel the stretch in your body.

Work Diamond into your evening routine. You may move into the stretch while you watch television or before you climb into bed, to ensure restful sleep.

## Number 4

Number 4 is a key stretch to practice every day. It helps lengthen the entire back of your body, from your heels to the back of your neck. It also strengthens your shoulders, arms, and torso while toning your abdomen, hips, and thighs.

**Flex Alert!** _____

If you suffer from sciatica or chronic back pain, omit this stretch from your routine and move on to Chapter 8.

1. Begin seated with your legs extended. Sit on a blanket if your back feels stiff. Place the sole of your right foot on your left inner thigh, bringing your right heel as close to your groin as you comfortably can while keeping your right knee on the floor. If you suffer from tight hamstrings, feel free to bend your extended knee. Your legs should be in the shape of the numeral 4. Rest your hands on the floor beside you, with your hips facing forward.

2. Glide your arms out to the sides and up, palms turned in as you inhale.

3. Slowly bend forward as you feel the back of your left leg and hamstring s-t-r-e-t-c-h. Exhale as you place your hands on either the ball of your foot, the top of your foot, or the ankle or shin of your left leg.

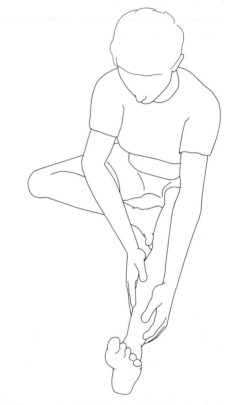

**Feel the stretch all along the back of your body with Number 4.**

4. Hold the stretch for four deep breaths while maintaining a flat back. Keep your chin tucked. As you inhale, feel your spine lengthen through the crown of your head. Use time and gravity to loosen tight muscles.

5. As you exhale, engage your abdominal muscles and round your torso over your left leg. Relax your upper body over your leg. Hold this position for four more breaths.

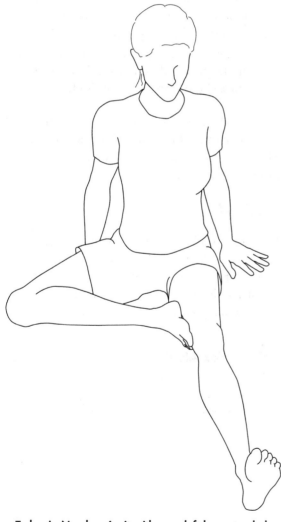

**To begin Number 4, sit with your left leg extended, your right foot on your left thigh, your heel in toward your groin, and your right knee on the floor.**

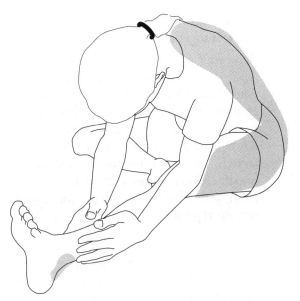

**As you exhale, relax your body over your leg.**

6. Move out of the stretch by raising your arms to your ears and then lifting your torso as you breathe in. Place your hands by your hips as you exhale, and pause to notice the difference between your right and left legs.

7. Extend your left leg straight and place your right foot on your inner left thigh, close to your groin. Repeat steps 1 through 6 on the other side of your body. Notice if you feel any difference on this side.

**Flex Alert!** _____

Don't lift your arms over your head if your back muscles are fragile or inflexible. Instead, rest your hands on the floor as you bring your torso back to a vertical position.

## Runner's Stretch

Here's a stretch you may already know by a different name: the lunge. Whatever you call it, this easy exercise is a classic hip opener. Keep your hips free and, as an added benefit, stretch the fronts of your thighs with the Runner's Stretch. As you hold this stretch and inhale, observe your spine lengthen toward the crown of your head.

1. On a soft surface or a mat or blanket, move to your hands and knees. Step your right foot forward between your hands, knee over your ankle, your shin straight. Extend your left leg backward, knee raised, toes rolled under so you're resting on the ball of your foot as you inhale.

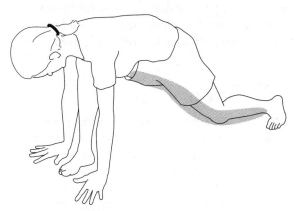

**Begin the Runner's Stretch with your right foot forward and your left leg back.**

**S-t-r-e-t-c-h It Out** _____

You may perform the lunge with your back knee down on a mat or blanket, if you need to. Place foam or wooden blocks under your hands if you need to raise the floor closer to you. See Appendix B for more on stretching resources and supplies.

2. Hold the stretch for four deep breaths, pressing your left heel back as you inhale. Press your hips toward the floor as you exhale. Gaze forward. You may bend your back knee to work your hip. Protect your vulnerable knees by keeping your right knee over your right ankle. Optimally, place your palms on either side of your front foot; if that doesn't work for you, make fists with your hands.

3. Move back to your hands and knees, and repeat steps 1 and 2 with your left leg forward and right leg back.

## Reclining Hip Flexor Stretch

This is a great stretch if you want to release tension after a long day, if you suffer from a tight back, or if you have been advised by a physician to stay off your feet or take it easy.

**Flex Alert!** _____

If you are more than 3 months pregnant, have recently undergone abdominal surgery, or suffer from serious back conditions, don't practice the Reclining Hip Flexor Stretch.

This stretch strengthens your lower back, stretches your *psoas muscles*, and improves leg and hip flexibility. In addition, your digestive system is stimulated from the pressure your leg and thigh exert on your colon.

**Flexicon** _____

Your **psoas muscles** are located on each side of your back. Chronically tight in most people, they originate at the spine around the bottom of the rib cage and run down to the pelvis and thigh bone.

1. Lie on your back, legs in a straight line and feet together. Inhale deeply.

2. Bend your right knee and draw it to your chest. As you exhale, clasp your hands on your shin, below your knee. Draw your chin toward your chest to lengthen the back of your neck. You may stretch your left leg along the floor to intensify the stretch. Remain in this position for four breaths, allowing your body to s-t-r-e-t-c-h, without force, as you become aware of your right hip.

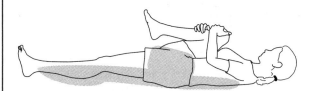

Feel the stretch in your hip and back as you lie on your back and hold your right knee toward your chest.

3. Slowly straighten your right leg and inhale as you move it back to the starting position. Exhale as you bend your left knee toward your chest. Follow the instructions in step 3 as you hold the stretch on this side of your body. Observe any differences on this side.

## Standing Hip Flexor Stretch

This standing stretch is a great way to start your day. It opens your hip and stretches your elusive psoas muscle. As an added benefit, it provides a nice stretch up your upper back and shoulder, and strengthens your arms and legs.

1. Stand steadily on a firm surface, with your feet even with your hips and your arms at your sides. Practice balance and coordination. Spreading your toes helps you establish a firm base of support. Gaze forward at one object to enhance your sense of balance.

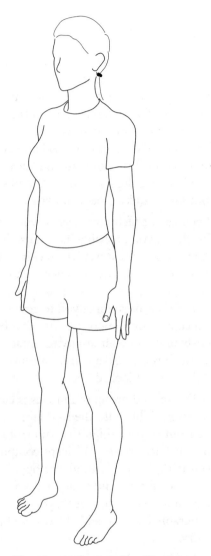

**Stand steadily to begin the Standing Hip Flexor Stretch, your feet hip-width apart and your arms at your sides.**

2. As you inhale, step forward with your right foot, about the length of your leg. Keep your feet even with your hips, your legs straight with a slight bend in your knees, and your weight placed evenly from front leg to back. Keep your feet flat on the floor and both hipbones facing forward. Rest your right hand lightly on your right thigh while your left arm rests by your side.

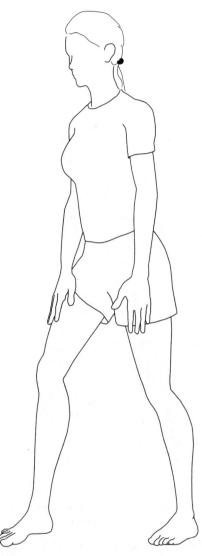

**Inhale and step your right foot forward, about a leg's length. Be sure to keep your balance.**

**S-t-r-e-t-c-h It Out**

Stand with both feet flat and firmly on the floor. You may swivel your left foot outward, if you need to, for balance.

3. Lift your left arm to your ear as you bend your right knee over your right ankle, leading with your chest, inhaling as you go. Pause here to s-t-r-e-t-c-h.

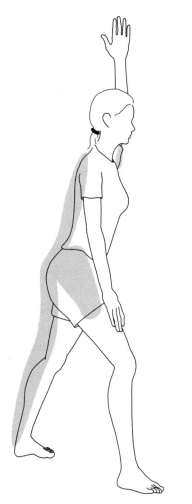

**Pause here to stretch, and feel it in your hip, back, and left arm.**

4. Exhale, straighten your right leg, and move your arm down by your side. Repeat this movement four times, remembering envelope breathing. As you move, keep your upper body relaxed to prevent tension in your back, shoulders, and neck.

5. Step your right foot back to the starting position, check your balance, and then step your left foot forward as you inhale, your left hand on your left thigh, your right arm at your side. Repeat the movements four times on this side of your body. Return to the starting position to pause, check your balance, and relax your breath.

# Stretching Your Legs

Your legs consist of two major muscle groups. The first group is known as the *hamstrings*. Running behind and below your knees, along the backs of your thighs, and all the way to your hips, your hamstrings serve a few important functions. They allow you to bend your knee joints, control the forward and backward movements of your legs as you walk, and stabilize your knees and legs as you twist.

If you can't touch your toes or you prefer slouching, you probably have tense hamstrings. Hamstring tension has far-reaching effects on your movement, your balance, and the health of your joints. Tight hamstrings restrict the extension of your hips, force you to round your back, and contribute to poor posture that can restrict movement and your ability to breathe. Stiff hamstrings are also a common cause of chronic back pain and locked knees.

The second group of muscles is called the *quadriceps*. These are the four large muscles at the front of your thigh that run from your hip to your knee. Your quadriceps complement your hamstrings by performing the opposite function: they extend and straighten your knees. If these muscles are too weak, you open up your vulnerable knees to added stress and potential injury.

And if your hamstrings are also too weak or inflexible, your quadriceps are prone to increased tension. That's why warming up and stretching both of these complementary muscle groups is essential to maintain their delicate balance and prevent strain or injury during exercise.

# Pyramid

Remember to practice your warm-ups before attempting leg stretches. Your legs will benefit from Pyramid as you increase flexibility and strength in your hamstrings, hips, and quadriceps. This asymmetrical stretch allows you to focus your attention on one side of your body at a time, which enables you to learn more about your body and how it works.

1. Stand on a firm surface, your feet even with your hips and your arms at your sides. Practice balance and coordination. Spreading your toes helps you establish a firm base of support. Gaze forward at one object to enhance your sense of balance.

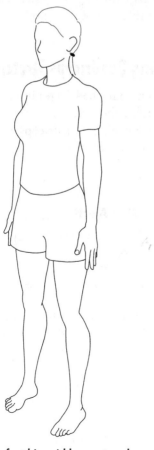

Stand with your feet hip-width apart and your arms at your sides.

2. Inhale as you step forward with your right foot, placing your right foot about a leg length in front of your left foot. Keep both legs straight with supple knees, feet flat on the floor, hips facing forward, weight even in both legs, arms by your sides.

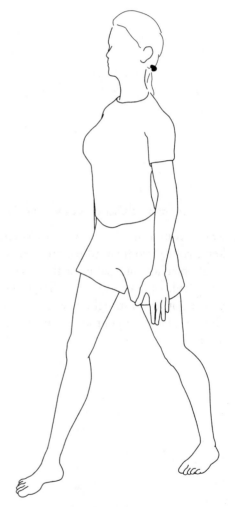

Step your right foot forward on your inhale, about a leg's length. Keep your feet hip-width apart, your arms by your sides.

3. Raise both arms out to your sides and up by your ears as you inhale, palms turned toward one another. Drop your shoulders away from your ears. Keep your joints and muscles relaxed, and use envelope breathing. Pause.

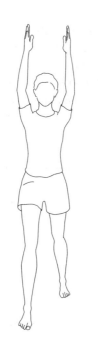

**Raise your arms to your ears as you inhale.**

4. Sweep your arms out to the sides as you bend your torso forward toward your right thigh, placing your palms or fingers on either side of your right foot. Try to keep your right leg as straight as you comfortably can, bending your knee only as needed. Your back leg should remain straight.

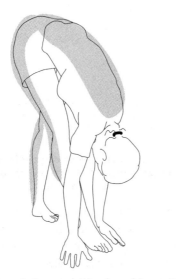

**Feel the stretch down your back and hamstrings as you lean forward.**

5. Sweep your arms out to the sides as you inhale up to your standing position, and exhale as you bend forward again, placing your hands by your front foot.

6. Repeat steps 3 and 4 two more times, ending in the forward bending position. Hold the stretch for four deep breaths. The hip of your back leg should press outward away from your spine.

7. To release the stretch, glide your arms out to the sides as you inhale your torso up, and bring both arms to your sides as you exhale. Pause to rest for a moment.

8. Perform the Pyramid on the other side of your body by placing your left leg forward and right leg back, proceeding through steps 1 through 7. Observe any differences on this side of your body.

## Kneeling Quadriceps Stretch

Lengthen your quadricep muscles, stretching your thighs, abdominal muscles, hips, and chest, with the Kneeling Quadriceps Stretch. You'll also hone your concentration skills and sense of balance.

**Flex Alert!** _____

Exclude the Kneeling Quadriceps Stretch from your routine if you have knee pain.

1. Start on your hands and knees. Bring your right foot forward, placing your right knee over your right ankle. Move your left knee directly under your left hip, placing your left knee on a folded blanket to protect it. Check your balance and then place your hands on top of your right knee. Avoid the tendency to lean on your bent knee; instead, lift your chest upward.

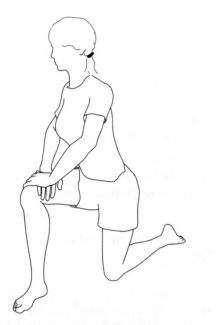

Begin the Kneeling Quadriceps Stretch with your right foot forward, your right knee over your right ankle, and your left leg back, with your left knee directly under your left hip.

2. Lunge forward with your right knee as you inhale deeply. Firm legs and a fixed forward gaze help you remain balanced and stable.

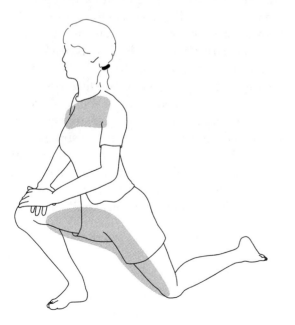

As you inhale, lunge forward.

3. Move back to the starting position as you exhale.

4. Glide back and forth three more times, inhaling as you move forward and exhaling as you move backward. Then hold the forward position for four breaths.

5. Practice the stretch on the other side of your body by placing your left foot forward and right leg back, as in step 1. Repeat steps 2 through 4.

## Standing Quadriceps Stretch

This routine elongates and loosens up your quads, keeping the front of your body long so you can stand erect, and reducing stress on your knees. Keep your shoulders even and engage your abdominal muscles as you practice this stretch. You'll walk and run with a longer, taller stride—almost as if you are gliding across the ground.

**S-t-r-e-t-c-h It Out**

Remember PNF (proprioceptive neuromuscular facilitation) stretching from Chapter 2? Try this effective technique in the Standing Quadriceps Stretch.

1. Stand tall, your feet even with your hips, your toes pointing forward. If it helps, steady yourself by holding on to a chair or placing your hand on a nearby wall.

2. Bend your right leg, and clasp your right foot with your right hand. Check your balance. Bring both knees toward one another, feeling the stretch in your right quadriceps.

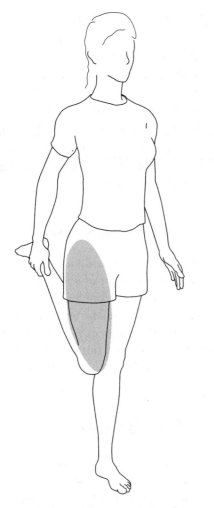

**Hold your right foot with your right hand. Keep your balance! (Use a chair or wall, if you need to.)**

3. Draw your ankle toward your buttocks Now create resistance by applying the PNF stretch: simultaneously press the top of your foot into your hand and press your hand into your foot. Hold for one long, deep breath; relax the press; and hold the stretch for four breaths without the PNF press.

**Flex Alert!** _____

Don't allow your knee to flare outward to the side. Keep your knees together.

4. Place your right foot back on the floor, and rest for three breaths.

5. Now stretch your right leg, repeating steps 1 through 4 two more times. Then stretch your left leg, repeating steps 1 through 4.

**A Stretch in Time ...** _____

You can practice the Standing Quadriceps Stretch anytime and anywhere. Try it right after your morning or evening shower when your muscles are pliable, or after walking or running for 5 minutes.

## Hamstring Stretch with Hands

The following supine stretches assist you in safely stretching your hamstrings and inner and outer thighs by using the floor to support your lower back. If you've had to skip stretches because of a sore back, this stretch is for you. The Hamstring Stretch with Hands helps you safely stretch the muscles at the back of your legs to prepare you for bending forward. If you make this stretch part of your daily routine, your back will thank you, as stretching the muscles and nerves in your hamstrings may prevent back problems, including sciatica. As an added benefit, you'll strengthen your abdominal muscles. You'll especially feel the results if you use the PNF technique in Chapter 2!

1. Lie on your back on a comfortable surface, feet close to your buttocks and even with your hips.

2. Inhale deeply, and as you exhale, raise your left leg, holding the back of your thigh. Keep your lower back flat on the floor as best you can. Flex your left foot, toes pointing toward your nose, and press your left heel toward the ceiling.

3. Continue to breathe as you slide your hands up your leg until you feel the back of your leg s-t-r-e-t-c-h. As you exhale, slide your hands up as far as you can to deeply stretch. Keep your foot flexed, inhale as you hold, reach through your heel, and exhale, remembering to engage your abdominal muscles.

4. To move even deeper into the stretch, inhale and s-t-r-e-t-c-h your right leg along the floor, pressing your left heel up toward the ceiling.

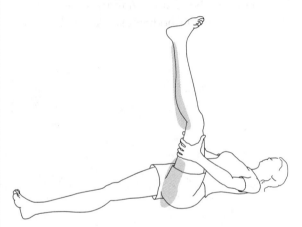

For a deeper stretch, extend your right leg along the floor.

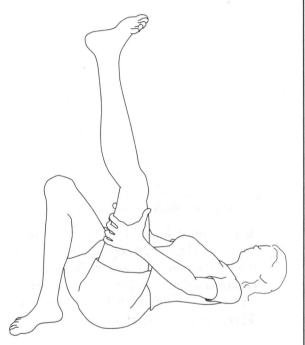

Lie on your back, and stretch that left leg up.

5. Once you've found just the right stretch for you, try applying the PNF technique: simultaneously press your leg into your hands and your hands into your leg for one breath. Then let go and stretch for four breaths. Practice this routine two more times.

6. Repeat steps 1 through 5, this time stretching your right leg.

### S-t-r-e-t-c-h It Out

If you can't hold the back of your leg with your hands, try using a strap, belt, or towel. Wrap the strap around the back of your left thigh, and hold the ends. Keep your shoulders as relaxed as possible.

# Inner Thigh Stretch

Another stretch accessible to those with tight backs, the Inner Thigh Stretch is performed in a supine (face up) position to stabilize your back. Often overlooked, your inner thigh muscles, or *adductors*, tend to be tight, especially after exercise. This routine releases tension in your hips and the muscles and nerve fibers in your groin. As an added benefit, it trims your hips, thighs, and abdominal muscles.

1. Start by lying on your back with your legs together. Move your arms out as you inhale so your body looks like the letter *T*.

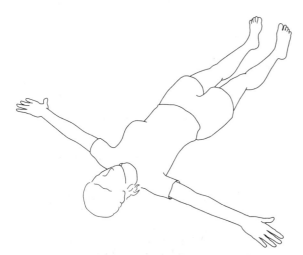

**Begin the Inner Thigh Stretch in the shape of the letter** T.

2. Exhale as you lift your left leg toward the sky. Press your left heel toward the ceiling as you inhale. Your right leg acts as an anchor during the stretch, so don't let your body tip.

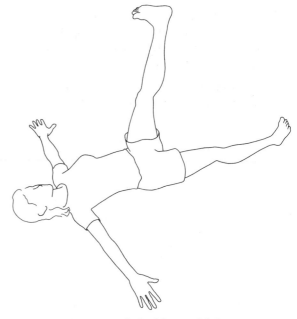

**On your exhale, lift your left leg.**

3. As you exhale, lower your left leg out to the left, and press the top of your right hip toward the floor with your right hand, to ensure you don't tip. Place your left hand on top of your left thigh, holding your hip down. Hold the stretch for four breaths.

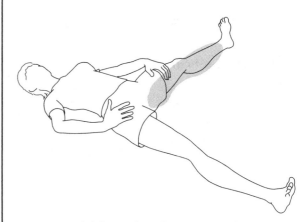

**Lower your left leg to the side, using your hands both for balance and to keep you from tipping.**

4. Repeat steps 2 and 3, this time stretching your right leg and your inner right thigh.

## Outer Thigh Stretch

This powerful stretch loosens your outer thigh muscles, or *abductors*, and a tough group of fibers called the *iliotibial* (IT) *bands*, which run along the outside of your thighs. Stiff outer thighs can cause a host of problems in your hips, knees, and back. Making this stretch a part of your routine prevents trouble; increases the range of motion in your hips and groin; and firms up abdominals, hips, and thighs. The supine position makes it safe for those with tight backs.

1. Start by lying on your back with your legs together. Move your arms out as you inhale so your body looks like the letter *T*.

2. Exhale and lift your left leg toward the sky at a 90-degree angle from your torso. Then inhale and press your left heel toward the ceiling.

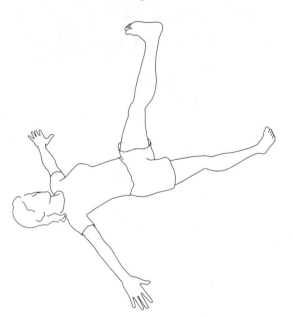

On your exhale, lift your left leg up into a 90-degree angle from your torso.

3. Exhale as you bring your left foot to the floor toward your right hand, and turn your head slowly to the left.

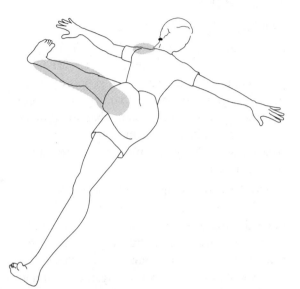

**Bring your left foot to the right and turn your head the opposite way. Feel the stretch in your outer thigh.**

4. With your left foot flexed, move your left leg toward the sky and inhale. Hold the twist for four breaths. Be sure you keep the left foot off the floor. If this causes strain, you can always use a strap for support. Keep your neck as relaxed as possible.

5. Repeat steps 3 and 4 three more times, remembering to breathe as you move.

6. To release the stretch, inhale as you lift your left leg, exhale as you hold it up, and inhale as you lower your left leg to meet your right leg.

7. Repeat steps 1 through 6, moving the right leg this time. Relax on your back and feel the effects of the stretch.

# Fabulous Feet, Knees, and Calves

Millions of people visit doctors every year because of foot and knee problems. If you don't want to be one of them, take time to care for your feet and lower legs, which support your upper body. Although these body parts are often ignored, stop and think about what you'd do without them. Basically, you would lose your balance, and a body out of balance suffers all sorts of misery.

Do you hear a snap, crackle, or pop from your knees when you bend or straighten them? Consider this a reminder: if you take care of your knees now, you might save yourself from years of pain. Each of your intricate knees consists of four joints, several ligaments, and a *meniscus*. These parts work together to let you bend, straighten, and rotate, all the while bearing your body weight. It's essential, then, to keep the muscles, tendons, ligaments, and joints that support your knees strong and flexible.

**Flexicon** _____

The **meniscus** is a crescent-shaped cartilage disc cushioning the end of a bone where it meets another bone in a joint, especially in the knee.

Have you ever been awakened by a muscle spasm in your calf? That's a clear sign that it's time to stretch your calves. They're an important group of muscles! Formed by the *gastrocnemius* and the *soleus*, your calves extend to your foot at the ankle and flex your toes, enabling you to jump, walk, run, and cycle. When you stretch your calf muscles, you help prevent injuries, and all other leg muscles will fall into place.

## On Your Toes

Wake up your feet, ankles, and calves by balancing On Your Toes. Balance, coordination, strength, and flexibility are the gifts you'll receive by making this stretch a part of your program. It's a good stretch to start with, as it helps you focus your attention on your body.

**Flex Alert!** _____

Those with injured feet, ankles, or calves should wait for a full recovery before trying this stretch. If you decide to proceed, you might want to support yourself with a nearby wall if you find it difficult to balance by yourself.

1. Stand with your feet and ankles together, arms at your sides for balance.

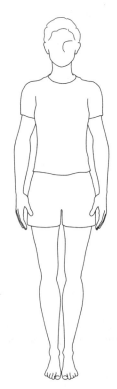

**Begin On Your Toes with your feet and ankle bones together, your arms at your sides.**

2. Inhale, and while still maintaining your balance, raise your heels until you feel a stretch. At the same time, raise your arms out to the sides and up over your head, palms together at the top. Pause. You can balance more easily when you stand on a flat surface. Focus your attention on one point at eye level, perhaps the horizon.

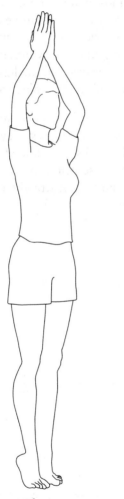

**Stand on your toes with your arms over your head, palms together.**

3. Slowly lower your heels and arms back to the starting position as you exhale.

4. Repeat steps 1 through 3 three more times. If you feel strong and steady, try holding step 2 for four breaths.

# Toe Tingler

All curled up in shoes most of the time, your toes are often immobile. Loosening them up through stretching can help relieve stiff joints associated with arthritis. Flexible toes also help you keep your balance. Once you've completed Toe Tinglers—moving your toes slowly and holding each position a few seconds—notice if your toes tingle and then move directly to Ankles Alive.

 **S-t-r-e-t-c-h It Out** _____

If sitting with your legs outstretched doesn't feel right, practice the Toe Tingler, Ankles Alive, and Ankle Circles lying on your back with your legs stretched toward the ceiling.

1. Sit with your legs outstretched and your feet slightly apart, hands somewhat behind your buttocks, on a folded blanket if you need to. Use your arms to support your back as you lean back a little.

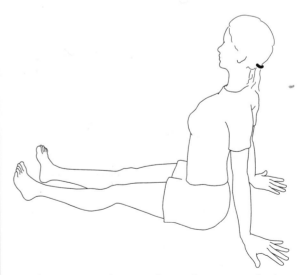

**To begin Toe Tingler, sit with your legs outstretched, your feet slightly apart, and your hands behind you, leaning back.**

2. With your feet flexed and your toes pointing toward the sky, focus your attention on your toes. Inhale and flex and spread your toes. Exhale and point and scrunch your toes.

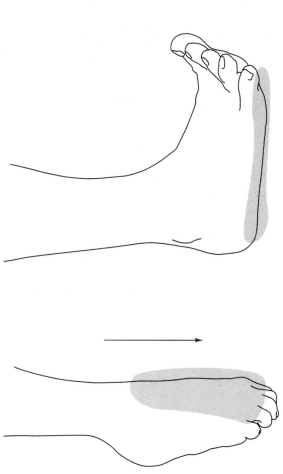

On your inhale, spread your toes and point them toward your nose. On your exhale, point your toes away and scrunch them.

3. Repeat step 2 nine more times. Focus your attention on the stretch sensations, your breathing, and your count.

## Ankles Alive

Your ankle is a large joint, capable of moving in two directions: away from your body and toward your body. Bones, ligaments, tendons, and muscles work together to move your ankle, which, in turn, moves your foot, providing you with the means to move your body. Ankle sprains, one of the most common musculoskeletal injuries, commonly occur when the muscles around your ankle are weak. Ankles Alive strengthens weak muscles, lubricates your ankle joint, and stretches your calves and the ligaments and tendons in your vulnerable ankle area.

1. Sit with your legs outstretched, your feet slightly apart, hands somewhat behind your buttocks, on a folded blanket if you need to. Use your arms to support your back, and keep it straight as you lean back a little.

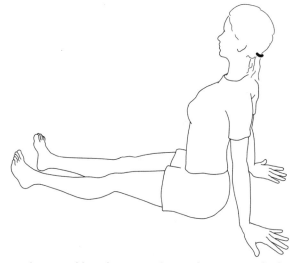

To begin Ankles Alive, sit with your legs outstretched, your feet slightly apart, and your hands behind you, leaning back.

2. With your feet flexed and toes pointing upward to start, inhale as you move your feet toward your nose. Exhale as you move your toes away from your nose. The challenge here is to keep your spine straight and your ankles relaxed and motionless as you stretch your toes.

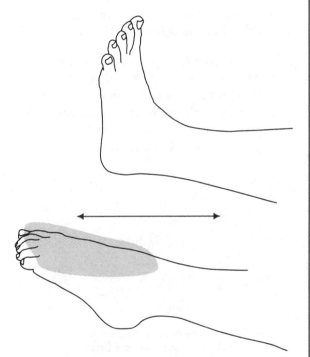

Inhale and bring your foot toward your nose. Exhale and point your foot away.

3. Repeat step 2 nine more times, holding each position for a few seconds.

## Ankle Circles

Once you've stretched your toes and loosened up your ankles, move on to Ankle Circles. As a complement to Ankles Alive, this stretch offers the same benefits. Don't be alarmed if you hear sounds as you move—that's just the natural sound of your ankle joint opening.

1. Sit with your legs outstretched, your feet slightly apart, and your hands somewhat behind your buttocks, on a folded blanket if you need to. Use your arms to support your back, and keep it straight as you lean back a little. Alternately, you can lie on your back with your legs raised.

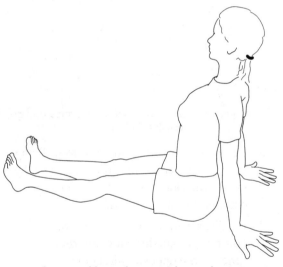

To begin Ankle Circles, sit with your legs outstretched, your feet slightly apart, and your hands behind you, leaning back.

2. Keep your legs separated but straight and your heels on the ground if you're sitting. Rotate your left foot clockwise 10 times and then counterclockwise 10 times. Inhale as you move your foot up, and exhale as you move it down. Pay close attention to the circling motion, closing your eyes to avoid distraction. Notice the range of motion in each ankle as you move.

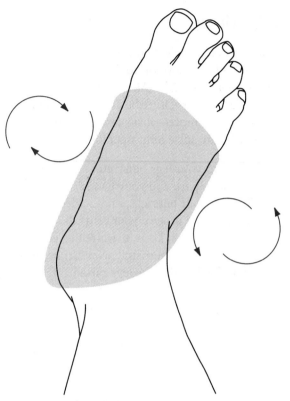

Rotate your foot clockwise, and then reverse and go counterclockwise.

3. Repeat step 2 with your right foot. Bring both feet together and rotate them at the same time clockwise 10 times and then counterclockwise 10 times.

4. Finally, separate your feet and rotate them 10 times in one direction and then 10 times in the opposite direction.

### S-t-r-e-t-c-h It Out

It's common to experience cramps in your feet once you begin to stretch them. If cramps occur, take a break from stretching and massage your foot. When the cramp subsides, resume your routine.

## Double Knee Bends

Gently move your knees—and give them a well-deserved break—without placing any pressure on your joints with Double Knee Bends. Your calves and the muscles surrounding your knees get stretched and strengthened, helping prevent knee strain or injury. This asymmetric stretch permits you to "take a look" at each knee and notice the differences between the two.

1. Lie on your back, your chin toward your chest, your knees bent, and your feet parallel on the floor and even with your hips. As you inhale, lift your left foot and, with your elbows bent, place your hands behind your left thigh by your knee. Exhale.

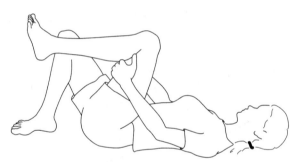

Begin Double Knee Bends on your back, with your chin toward your chest and your feet on the floor, parallel and hip-width apart. Bring your left foot up as you inhale.

2. Straighten your left leg as you inhale, flexing your foot toward the ceiling but keeping your knee slightly bent and your arms straight. Keep your lower back flat on the floor.

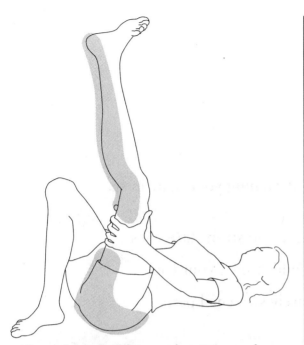

**Lift your left leg and flex your foot. Be sure to keep your lower back flat on the floor.**

3. Return to the starting position as you exhale.

4. Repeat steps 1 through 3, this time placing your hands behind your right thigh by your knee.

5. Alternate, stretching your right and left legs a total of 12 times.

## The Least You Need to Know

◆ Maintaining a strong and flexible base reduces the effects of gravity over time, allows your spine to lengthen upward, and enables you to breathe easily.

◆ Letting your upper body open and expand increases flexibility in your spine and hips.

◆ Lack of elasticity in your hamstrings and hips inhibits your ability to bend forward, thus creating a tight back.

◆ Forgetting to stretch your quadriceps and your inner and outer thigh muscles can lead to leg, hip, and lower-back problems.

◆ Although you seldom pay attention to your feet, knees, and calves, it's essential to perform exercises to stretch and strengthen your vital foundation.

# In This Chapter

- ◆ Discover the benefits of stretching your body in six directions
- ◆ Distinguish between gentle and strong stretches
- ◆ Understand why you should stretch your back
- ◆ Learn to stretch those rarely stretched parts

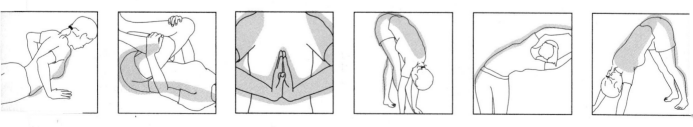

# Stretching Your Whole Body

Your body was created to stay in perfect balance, but time and age can bring on challenges. So keeping yourself healthy, strong, and flexible is a great general health check. Remember, you were created to function with ease. Stretching your body fine-tunes your system, allowing your flexible body to adapt as you maneuver along the bumps on life's road.

In this chapter, you consolidate all you've learned about stretching your body and apply these principles as you stretch. Once you learn and memorize just six key movements ...

1. Bending backward
2. Bending forward
3. Stretching to your right side
4. Stretching to your left side
5. Twisting your body to the right
6. Twisting your body to the left

... you'll have a straightforward, intelligent system for stretching your whole body. These six directional stretches keep your body balanced and strong. Soon you'll discover that your new stretching habit works like magic, as aches and pains progressively disappear.

Practicing whole-body stretches provides a necessary warm-up and an essential cool-down to vigorous activity to prevent injuries and keep muscles supple. These essential stretches keep your muscles and connective tissue healthy and flexible. You'll prevent and treat sore muscles, nourish your joints and spine, and feel relaxed and renewed as you release muscle tension.

# Gentle Stretches

Gentle stretches balance the effects of repetitive movements or the tightness that appears in the body after remaining in one position for an extended period of time. Use them to release stress at the end of the day or to stretch stiff muscles when you wake up in the morning. Stretching your muscles gently helps calm your mind as you release tension.

Although everyone can practice these gentle stretches, they are especially beneficial for those with weak, strained, tender, or tight muscles that need to be lightly stretched. Gentle stretches are a great way to warm up before exercising or as a precursor to the later strong stretches, and those new to stretching should also start here. Allowing your body to ease into a stretching routine is wise.

Keep your muscles and joints relaxed and soft as you stretch. Move slowly to open up your body. Don't forget to breathe deeply.

## Receiving Stretch

Everyone can practice the Receiving Stretch. Counteracting the tension in your neck, shoulders, and upper back, your challenge here is to keep your muscles and joints *relaxed* as you stretch. Stretching your body in this manner loosens vertebrae. This relaxed stretch balances the effects of habitually rounding your upper back forward as you perform daily tasks—and hiking your shoulders up toward your ears as you brace yourself. You will breathe easier if you master the Receiving Stretch and make it a part of your morning routine. It's so easy.

1. Stand with your arms at your sides, your feet hip-width apart. Close your eyes for a moment, if you feel steady, and relax.

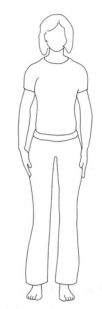

Start the Receiving Stretch standing with your arms at your sides and your feet hip-width apart.

2. S-t-r-e-t-c-h your arms out to your sides and up over your head, inhaling as you move.

3. Look up at your palms as they come together. Relax your shoulders. Pause.

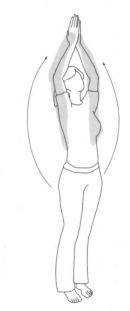

Raise your arms over your head, bringing your palms like in a prayer, and look up.

4. Exhale. Allow your arms to float back down to your sides. Pause.

5. Repeat these movements two more times.

### S-t-r-e-t-c-h It Out

Remember envelope breathing (from Chapter 2). Always "envelop" your movements with breath. As you stretch, breathe into your stretch.

## Gentle Side Stretch

Stretching your sides isn't the most common of stretches, which makes it that much more of an essential part of your stretching routine. Enter each stretch slowly and carefully. You may also place your hands on your hips rather than raising your arms over your head, if that feels more comfortable. Stand straight and tall after stretching one side of your body. Notice if you can feel a difference between the stretched side and the side waiting to be stretched. Once your side stretching is complete, close your eyes, if you're steady, and feel both sides of your body. Both sides should feel strengthened, toned, and balanced.

1. Start by standing with your feet hip-width apart, arms by your sides.

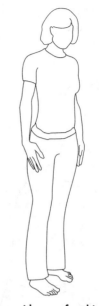

Begin by standing with your feet hip-width apart and your arms by your sides.

2. Sweep your left arm up by your ear, palm turned in, inhaling as you go. S-t-r-e-t-c-h.

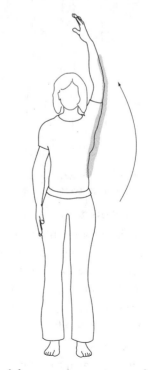

Stretch your left arm up by your ear, palm turned in, while your right arm rests by your side.

3. Bend, gliding your hips to the left and your torso to the right, as you exhale. Gaze forward.

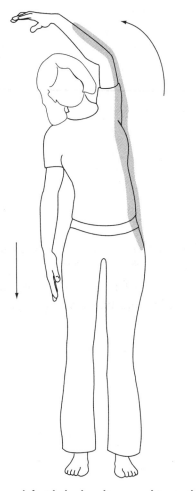

Stretch your left side by bending your hips to the left and your torso to the right.

4. Repeat the movements two more times.

5. Finally, hold the stretch four long inhales and exhales, engaging the core of your body as you exhale to protect your back. Do not twist, and keep your gaze forward.

6. Slowly lift your left arm and torso as you inhale. Lower your left arm to your side, exhaling as you go. Stand straight.

7. Raise your right arm to your ear, palm turned in, inhaling as you s-t-r-e-t-c-h.

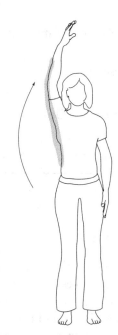

Raise your right arm up by your ear, palm turned in, while your left arm rests by your side.

8. Bend, gliding your hips to the right and your torso to the left, as you exhale. Look forward.

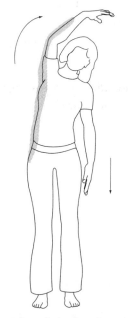

Stretch your right side by bending your hips to the right and your torso to the left.

9. Repeat the stretch two more times.

10. Hold the stretch for four deep breaths, moving deeper into the side stretch.

11. To release the stretch, slowly lift your right arm and torso as you inhale. Exhale and lower your right arm to your side, to standing. Notice how each side of your body feels.

## Gentle Twist

Twisting acts as a massage for your insides, compressing and stretching your abdominal organs. Let go of mental and physical tensions as you stretch. Move slowly and carefully as you release toxins from your body. You'll unwind and feel light.

Do not twist if your back is injured or inflamed. And check your balance—it's important to keep your weight evenly distributed in each foot during the twist. Do not lean to the side, but keep your feet firmly planted.

1. Stand, feet hip-width apart, with your hands on your hips. Inhale.

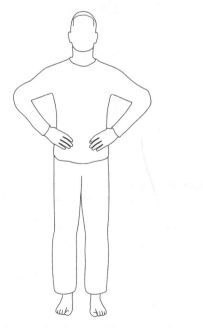

Stand with your feet hips-width apart with your hands on your hips.

2. Twist your torso to the right, looking over your right shoulder, exhaling as you twist. Pause to feel the twist.

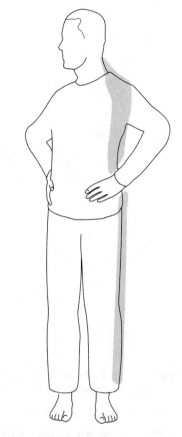

Stand with your feet hip-width apart and your hands on your hips. Twist your torso to the right.

3. Unwind to center as you inhale.

4. Repeat the twist as you exhale, turning a little deeper.

5. Inhale as you unwind.

6. Repeat these movements one more time.

7. Remain in the twist for four long inhales and exhales.

8. Unwind as you inhale and come back to the starting position.

9. Now twist your torso to the left, looking over your left shoulder, exhaling as you move.

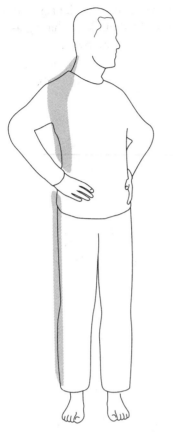

Stand with your feet hip-width apart with your hands on your hips. Twist your torso to the left.

10. Unwind to center as you inhale.

11. Repeat the twist as you exhale, turning a little deeper.

12. Inhale as you unwind.

13. Repeat these movements one more time.

14. Hold the twist for four long breaths.

15. Release the stretch as you breathe in.

16. Exhale. Relax your arms beside your body and feel the effects of the twist.

## Gentle Half Back Stretch

Stretching your back with the Gentle Half Back Stretch helps counteract your back's natural tendency to tighten as you age.

Do not attempt this or the Gentle Full Back stretches if your back is sore or injured, or if you have sciatic pain. Bend your knees if you feel any tightness or strain in your lower back.

1. Stand with your feet hip-width apart. Let your arms hang at rest beside your body.

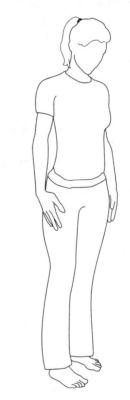

Stand, placing your feet hip-width apart, and allowing your arms to relax beside your body.

2. Sweep your arms to the sides and up over your head as you breathe in. Look up at your fingers as they lightly touch. Drop your shoulders away from your ears. Pause for a moment.

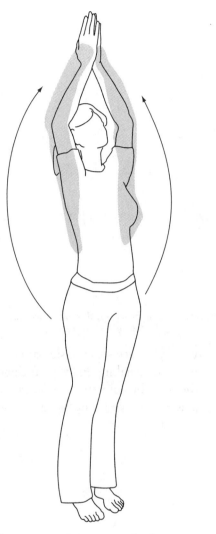

**Standing, sweep your arms up. Look up to your hands as your fingers touch.**

3. Glide your arms out to the sides, exhaling. Lead with your arms—not your chin—as you bend your knees slightly, and slowly bend forward, placing your torso halfway up. Your back should be straight as a table. Keep your arms out to the sides, your elbows slightly bent. Pause.

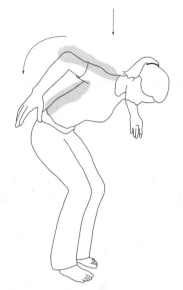

**Leading with your arms, slowly bend forward. That's enough, just halfway, with your knees bent.**

4. Inhale your body back to standing, arms stretched over your head.

5. Fold again as you exhale.

6. Repeat steps 1 through 5 again and hold the half-forward bend four long breaths, chin toward chest, *flat back*. If your back and arms become tired, place your hands on your thighs, but keep your back flat.

### Flexicon

**Flat back** means that your back is as flat as a table. With time and practice, you'll be able to feel the difference between a flat back and a rounded back. Try this stretch by a mirror to check for a flat back.

7. After the third exhale, s-t-r-e-t-c-h your arms to your sides, raising your torso to the standing position.

8. Bring your arms to your sides as you exhale. Relax.

# Gentle Full Back Stretch

Stretch, strengthen, and tone the back and the front of your body with Gentle Full Back Stretch. Bend your knees as much as you need to place your fingers by your toes. Soften your knees and neck as you go. Bend from your hips, not your waist. Focus on what you are doing as you practice this stretch.

1. Start standing, your feet hip-width apart with your chin tucked toward your chest.

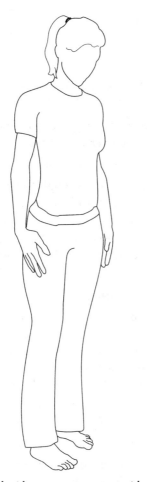

**Stand with your arms at your sides.**

2. S-t-r-e-t-c-h your arms to the side and up as you breathe in. Gaze upward at your touching fingertips.

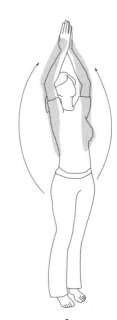

**Stand with your arms up, fingers touching, your gaze to your fingertips.**

3. Float your arms to the side as you bend forward, exhaling. Place your fingers on the floor by your toes, if you can, and pause. Bend your knees slightly, if you have to.

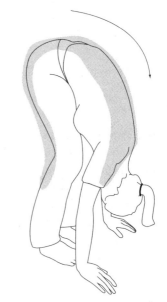

**Bend forward and place your fingers by your toes. Slightly bend your knees if you need to.**

4. Sweep your arms out, lift your torso back to standing with your arms stretched upward, and inhale.

5. Bend forward again as you exhale.

6. Repeat this sequence three times and then hold the full back stretch four long breaths.

7. S-t-r-e-t-c-h your arms out to the sides, lift your torso back to standing, and stretch your arms over your head as you inhale.

8. Exhale your arms to your sides.

**S-t-r-e-t-c-h It Out** _____

Practice each sequence of stretches in order; don't skip to the strongest stretch right away. Treat each initial stretch as a warm-up, and ease into the next stretch in the sequence.

# Strong Stretches

The strong stretches here are a powerful routine to strengthen your muscles and make you feel solid and healthy. With experience, you'll come to enjoy the feeling of release that accompanies each stretch.

Moving and holding these strong stretches can be vigorous and intense. Warm up beforehand by practicing the warm-up stretches in Chapter 2, by doing the gentle stretches earlier in this chapter, or by walking or jogging for 5 to 10 minutes. Position your body to receive the maximum stretch, but remember: don't go past your edge. You'll enjoy stretching stronger and longer if you don't force or strain.

Because these strong stretches invigorate your body, try not to schedule them as a nighttime routine. Instead, practice them when you rise in the morning to wake up sleepy muscles, during a break in your day to energize your

body, or after exercising to reduce muscle soreness. As always, don't forget to breathe deeply as you stretch.

## Shoulder and Chest Expander

Keep your shoulder joints flexible with the Shoulder and Chest Expander stretch. Shoulder inflexibility is a common problem. Most people lose their full range of shoulder rotation as they age. This stretch helps preserve the flexibility of this healthy, intricate joint, maintaining your ability to rotate your shoulders and arms. It is one of the most important stretches in this chapter and one you should master.

1. Stand, feet hip-width apart, chin to chest.

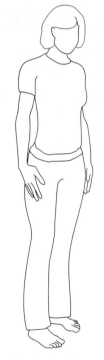

Stand with your feet hip-width apart and your chin tucked.

2. S-t-r-e-t-c-h your arms out to the sides and up as you inhale.

3. Interlace your fingers, press your palms up, and s-t-r-e-t-c-h.

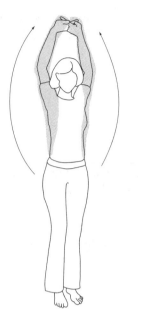

**Stand with your arms up, and interlace your fingers for an added stretch.**

4. Lean back and sweep your arms out, palms up, exhaling.

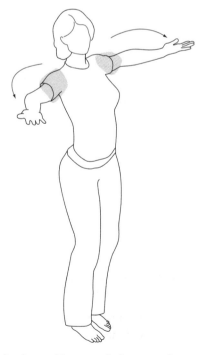

**Lean back watching your balance, and sweep your arms out and then forward.**

5. End standing straight, your arms stretched forward, your palms upward.

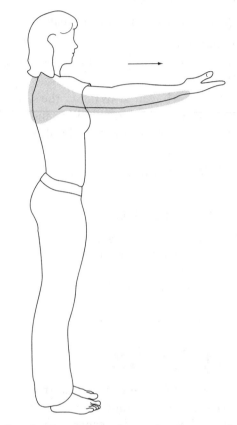

**Stand with your arms forward, palms turned up.**

**Flex Alert!** _____

Sore backs stop here. Remember, bend your knees before you lean back, to protect your back. Let your back's muscles be your guide.

6. Again, lean back and sweep your arms out, palms up, as you inhale.

7. End standing straight, your arms stretched over your head. Interlace your fingers, press your palms up, and s-t-r-e-t-c-h.

8. S-t-r-e-t-c-h your arms out to the sides and down, exhaling. Pause.

9. Practice steps 1 through 6 two more times.

# Strong Side Stretch

Regularly performing this stretch keeps your spine supple and strengthens the central part of your body, especially your abdomen, where you'll stimulate the digestive, circulatory, and respiratory systems.

First practice the Strong Side Stretch moving from side to side regularly for approximately 1 month before you attempt to hold the stretch. Be sure you don't twist your spine, do look forward at all times, and keep your upper shoulder rolled back.

1. Stand with your feet and anklebones together, your chin tucked.

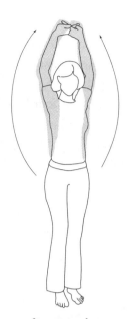

Interlace your fingers and press your palms to the sky.

3. Sway to the right, exhaling as you go. Feel a nice stretch up the left side of your body.

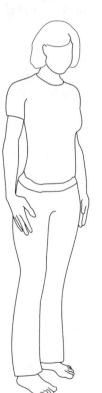

Stand with your feet together, chin tucked, and arms to your sides.

2. Sweep both arms out to your sides, inhaling as you stretch. Interlace your fingers, press your palms skyward, and s-t-r-e-t-c-h.

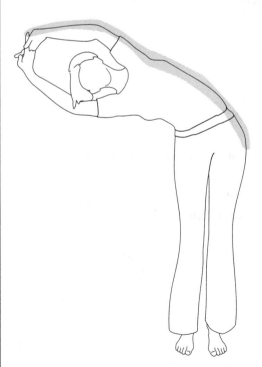

Bend to the right with your fingers interlaced and your arms extended.

4. Inhale back to standing.

5. S-t-r-e-t-c-h your side again as you exhale.

6. Repeat these movements one more time, stretching right.

7. Hold the stretch for four long breaths.

8. Inhale back to standing.

9. Sway your body to the left. Exhale as you s-t-r-e-t-c-h.

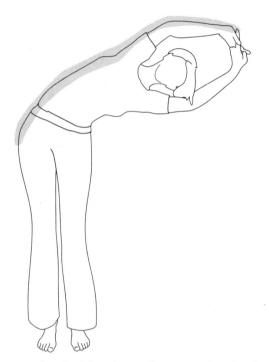

**Bend to the left with your fingers interlaced and your arms extended.**

10. Inhale back to standing.

11. Stretch your side again as you exhale.

12. Repeat the stretch one more time, then hold the stretch for four long breaths.

13. Inhale back to standing.

14. Exhale and lower both arms to your sides. Pause to feel the effects of the work.

# Strong Twist

Twisting movements keep your structure in harmony, bringing strength, flexibility, and life to your spine. Feel free to try the Strong Twist if you're healthy and strong and have no back pain. You'll realign your spinal column at the same time that you loosen your back.

Twisting gives your internal organs a gentle massage, and over time, your abdomen will become strong and trim with this stretch. Deepen the twist as you strongly exhale. Check your balance and keep your weight even. Intensify the stretch with each repetition. You'll love the results.

1. Stand, feet together and chin tucked.

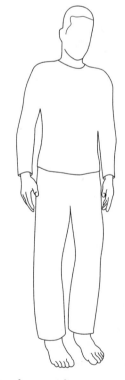

**Stand with your feet together, arms to your sides and tuck your chin.**

2. S-t-r-e-t-c-h your arms out to the sides and up over your head, inhaling as you move.

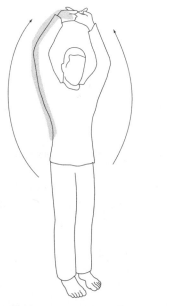

**Feel the stretch in your arms. Your fingers are interlaced and palms up.**

3. Twist your torso to the right, looking over your right shoulder, exhaling as you twist.

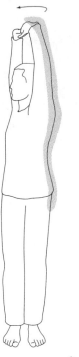

**Stand with your arms up, your fingers interlaced, your palms up. Twist your torso to the right.**

4. Inhale and release the twist.

5. Repeat the twist, exhaling as you go. Turn a little deeper this time, if you can.

6. Inhale and unwind.

7. Repeat these movements one more time.

8. Hold the twist for four breaths, lengthening your spine as you inhale. Deepen the twist as you exhale.

9. Come back to center as you inhale.

10. Exhale as you release your fingers and arms back to your sides.

11. Raise your arms out and up, interlacing your fingers at the top and inhaling as you s-t-r-e-t-c-h.

12. This time twist to the left, looking over your left shoulder, exhaling as you go.

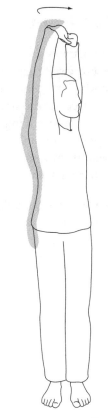

**Stand with your arms up, your fingers interlaced, and your palms up. Twist your torso to the left.**

13. Release the twist, inhaling as you move.
14. Repeat the twist as you exhale.
15. Move out of the twist as you breathe in and twist again, exhaling as you s-t-r-e-t-c-h.
16. Remain in the strong twist four long, smooth breaths.
17. Inhale back to center.
18. Lower your arms as you breathe out.

**Flex Alert!**

If you feel pain when you twist, stop stretching and consult a doctor. If you find it hard to breathe in the twist, feel free to open your mouth.

## Strong Half Back Stretch

Consulting your doctor is always wise before starting any new exercise program, stretching included. Those who have practiced the gentle stretches for a few weeks, who have healthy backs, and/or who have stretching experience will benefit the most from this strong stretch. Remember to bend from your hips, *not* your waist, and keep your back flat.

1. Stand with your feet and anklebones together, your chin tucked.

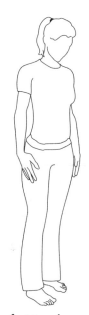

Stand with your feet together, your arms to your sides your chin tucked.

2. Sweep your arms out and up, inhaling as you go. Interlace your fingers, press your palms up, and s-t-r-e-t-c-h.

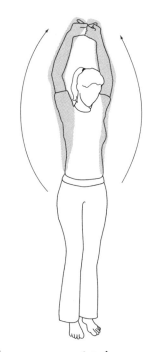

Stand with your arms up, interlace your fingers, and turn your palms up.

3. Exhale and bend halfway forward, fingers interlaced, flat back, hinging from your hips. Keep your arms by your ears and your chin to your chest.

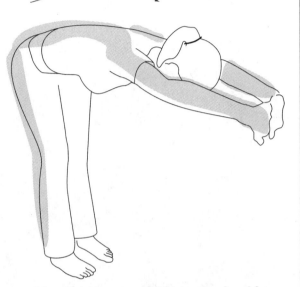

Bend forward, arms out, and fingers interlaced for a that extra-special stretch.

4. Lift your torso to standing, inhaling as you move. Exhale and bend halfway forward. Repeat these movements one more time.

5. Now hold the half back stretch for four long inhales and exhales.

6. Straighten your torso to standing. Release your arms to your sides.

## Strong Full Back Stretch

This intense stretch improves circulation to all the major muscle groups and, thus, strengthens and tones your thighs, calves, gluteal muscles, and back—those muscles hard to access and keep fit. It strengthens your abdomen muscles, too. Holding this stretch increases blood flow to your brain, calming your mind and adding vitality to your life. That's a lot for one stretch!

1. Stand with your feet and anklebones together, your chin tucked.

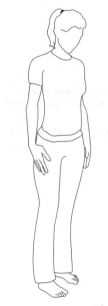

Stand with your arms to your sides, your chin to your chest.

2. S-t-r-e-t-c-h your arms out and up. Inhale. Interlace your fingers, press your palms up, and s-t-r-e-t-c-h.

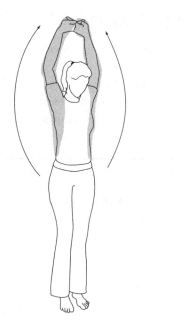

**Stretch your arms up, fingers interlaced, and press your palms up. Breathe.**

3. Release your fingers, and face your palms forward.

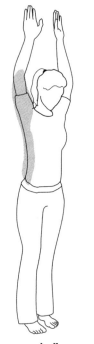

**Release your fingers and allow your palms to turn forward.**

4. Bend forward, hinging from the hips, exhaling as you move. Keep your back flat. Imagine that an object you want to touch is just beyond your reach. Place your hands by your feet, bending your knees, if needed.

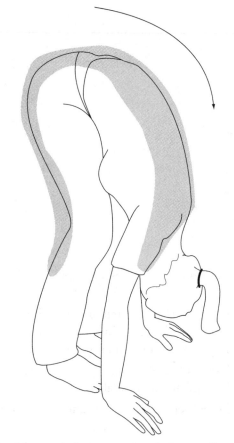

**Bend forward placing your hands by your feet. It's okay to bend your knees.**

5. Raise your arms to your ears and interlace your fingers. Now lift your torso and really s-t-r-e-t-c-h as you inhale.

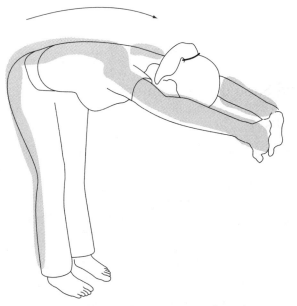

**Bend forward. Extend your arms and interlace your fingers.**

6. Release your fingers, face your palms forward, and dive again, exhaling as you go.

7. Repeat these movements one more time. Move with your breath.

8. Now hold the Strong Full Back Stretch four long inhales and exhales.

9. Inhale and lift your arms to your ears. Interlace your fingers. Press your palms away. Inhale as you move to a standing position.

10. Lower your arms to your sides as you exhale.

**A Stretch in Time ...**

Bending forward calms your mind. Use the Strong Full Back Stretch anytime you need to release stress. While holding the stretch, consciously let go of anything that no longer serves you.

## The Least You Need to Know

◆ Stretching your body six ways—bending backward and forward, stretching to the right and to the left, and twisting to the right and left—keeps your muscles and connective tissue healthy and flexible, and lubricates your joints.

◆ Opening the front of your body prevents your shoulders from rounding.

◆ Stretching your back helps counteract the natural tendency of your back to tighten as you age.

◆ Stretching your sides is an essential part of your routine.

◆ Twisting releases toxins from your body and gives your internal organs a gentle massage.

# In This Part

6 Relieving Head, Neck, and Shoulder Discomfort

7 Easing Joint Pain and Stiffness

8 Sore Backs Stop Here

9 Sports Stretching

10 Seniors' Stretch

11 Just for Her

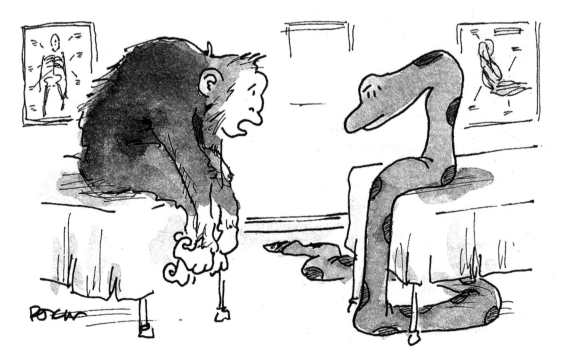

*"Yeah, my back is killing me, too."*

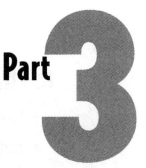

# Part 3

# Niche Stretching: Customizing Your Routine

Part 3 offers customized stretching routines to meet your specific, personal needs. Stretches for common aches and pains are summarized so you'll know where to turn when discomfort arises. Once you're well, enhance your favorite sport as you practice sport-specific stretching routines. Seniors explore how to maintain strength, flexibility, and balance—reducing chances of illness and injury and women will have no excuse but to pamper themselves with special stretches designed to help you relax into all the stages of your life with grace and master quick and easy stress-relieving techniques to keep you healthy.

## In This Chapter

- ◆ Ease headaches
- ◆ Release jaw tension
- ◆ Nurse your neck with stretch therapy
- ◆ Lift the weight off your shoulders

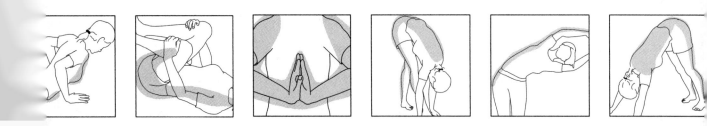

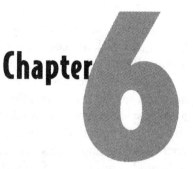

# Relieving Head, Neck, and Shoulder Discomfort

In this and the following chapters, we guide you as you embark on a stretch treatment plan tailor-made to meet your unique needs. We explore some important do's and don'ts, causes and symptoms, and benefits and contraindications along the way, too.

Rediscover the joy of living by gradually reducing or eliminating head, neck, and shoulder discomfort with the nine easy stretches in this chapter. As you explore the delicate relationship between your head, neck, shoulders, and spine, you'll empower yourself with concrete tools to address your particular concerns.

In the following pages, we share with you the knowledge you need to reduce or eliminate common reasons for headaches and pain in your jaw, neck, and shoulders. You'll find stretch prescriptions for common conditions such as TMJD (temporomandibular joint disorder) and frozen shoulder that pay particular attention to stretching techniques. When head, neck, or shoulder pain appears, you'll be ready to act, armed with your toolbox of stretches and tips.

By mastering the stretches in this chapter, you'll develop the body awareness you need to discover habitual movement patterns that may add to the causes of your pain or tension. You'll also explore ways to fine-tune your posture, practice breathing and relaxation techniques, and discover how and when to ward off headaches. Plus, you may improve the quality of your life as you increase your range of motion and reduce stress.

# Reverse Gravity to Cure Headaches

Headaches are most commonly caused by stress, hunger, and lack of sleep—three common conditions. Poor posture, such as rounded shoulders, a curved upper back, or a thrust-forward head can result in tense muscles and head pain, too. Muscle tension in the back of your neck and at the connection between your head and your neck and upper-back muscles can radiate to behind your eyes and forehead. And because muscle tension can cause headaches, stretching every day can prevent and treat this common and often debilitating affliction.

Soothe your pulsating brain and relax the back of your neck by positioning your heart above your head. You'll reverse the action of gravity on your body; instead of blood being pulled toward your feet, you'll shift it toward your head, encouraging a rich supply of blood to flow to your brain, relieving your headache and helping you concentrate.

**S-t-r-e-t-c-h It Out**

Start stretching at the first sign of pain, before your muscles contract.

The following Heels Over Head and A Frame stretches encourage correct posture, proper breathing, and relaxation, helping release the tension in your neck, shoulders, and upper back that commonly cause headaches. What are you waiting for?

## Heels Over Head Stretch

Here's a cure to unlock the vise grip of a tension headache. Move into this reclining stretch at the first sign of pain, and fall "head over heels" as you stretch away muscle tension while nourishing your facial skin, scalp, and hair roots. And as your venous circulation improves, you may also prevent varicose veins, because this restorative stretch allows blood and fluids that usually pool in your legs and trunk to flow toward your heart.

Skip this stretch if you have uncontrolled high or low blood pressure; chronic nasal, sinus, or thyroid disorders; or any infection or inflammation of your eyes or ears.

1. Lie on your right side, close to a wall, with your knees bent toward your chest. Scoot your hips so your feet and buttocks touch the wall.

Lie on your right side with your knees bent, your feet and buttocks touching the wall.

2. Roll to the left, swinging your legs up the wall. Open your arms from your shoulders out to the sides, palms up. If you feel tension in the backs of your legs, turn your legs slightly in and release any tightness in your knees.

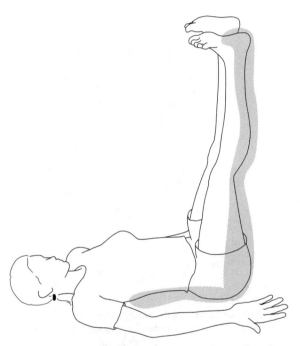

Lie on your back, with your legs up the wall and your arms stretched out.

3. Relax into the stretch and breathe deeply, holding the position at least 5 minutes. Your breathing should become slow and deep as you hold the stretch, relieving stress and relaxing muscles in your forehead, eyes, jaw, and tongue.

4. Come out of the stretch, retracing the steps you took to move into it. Bend your knees, roll to your side, and use your strong arms to move to your hands and knees. Place one foot on the floor, with your knee bent, and hold on to a chair or the wall for support as you raise your body to standing.

**Flex Alert!** _____

Prevent back strain by making sure your buttocks touch the wall. Tight hamstrings? Bend your knees as much as necessary to alleviate any pulling sensations in the backs of your legs.

## A Frame Stretch

When it feels like a boa constrictor of stress has crept up your shoulders, circled your neck, and encased your skull, causing a tension headache, move into the A Frame Stretch to soothe your pulsating brain. While you're at it, you'll also lengthen your spinal column; increase the flow of oxygen to your brain; expand your chest; strengthen and tone your abdomen, hips, and thighs; stretch the muscles and nerves in the back of your legs; and increase circulation.

Don't practice this stretch if you have uncontrolled high blood pressure, infection, or inflammation of the eyes or ears, or chronic injury or inflammation of your back, legs, ankles, knees, hips, wrists, arms, or shoulders.

**S-t-r-e-t-c-h It Out** _____

The A Frame Stretch requires a measure of strength and flexibility. Hold the stretch progressively longer to allow your body time to adjust to its strength. Bring your knees down and take breaks when you need to. If you experience pain, practice the Heels Over Head Stretch instead.

1. Move to your hands and knees, with your hands below your shoulders, your fingers spread, and your knees under your hips. Keep your shins and the tops of your feet on the floor. Kneel on a folded blanket to protect your knees, if you prefer.

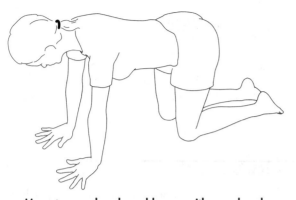

**Move to your hands and knees, with your hands beneath your shoulders and your knees under your hips.**

2. Curl your toes, spread your fingers wide apart, and inhale deeply into your chest. Exhale as you press into your hands and feet and lift your hips. Keep your neck muscles relaxed and your knees bent. Keep breathing deeply. Hold this stretch for a few breaths, to allow your body to adjust to this position.

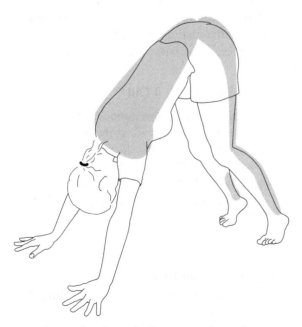

**With your hands on the floor, spread your fingers wide, curl your toes under, keep your hips up, and bend your knees.**

3. Inhale, bend your right knee and exhale, press your left heel toward the floor. Inhale as you bend your left knee and exhale press your right heel toward the floor. Alternate these movements six to eight times.

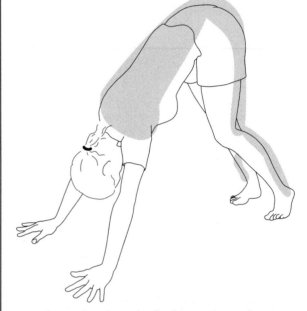

**With your hands on the floor, spread your fingers wide, curl your toes under, keep your hips up, and bend your left knee.**

4. Bring your knees to the floor as in step 1, and take a break.

5. Repeat step 2, moving back into the stretch, holding it and breathing deeply for four breaths, if possible. Don't force or strain. Gradually work toward holding the A Frame Stretch for six to eight breaths. Remember to keep your head and neck relaxed.

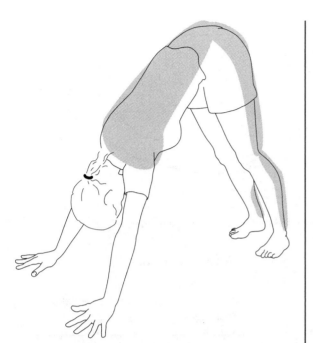

**Your hands on the floor with your fingers spread wide, your feet on the floor, and your hips up.**

# Temporomandibular Joint Disorder (TMJD)

Have you ever awakened with a sore jaw? Perhaps daily stresses and strains are causing you to clench your jaw at night, or maybe you're also tensing your jaw throughout the day. The cumulative effect of jaw tensing and teeth grinding may cause you to suffer from symptoms of *temporomandibular joint disorder*, commonly referred to as *TMJ* or *TMJD*.

Your temporomandibular joint is found at the point where your lower jaw meets the *temporal bone* of your skull. You can find it right in front of each ear on the side of your head. One of the most frequently used joints in your body, this intricate joint moves every time you swallow

and talk. Consequently, if you've been diagnosed with temporomandibular joint disorder, you may be experiencing frequent discomfort.

> ### Flexicon
> **Temporomandibular joint disorder** is a variety of conditions that cause pain and discomfort in the temporomandibular joint where your lower jawbone joins the temporal bone of your skull. Your **temporal bones** consist of five parts and are found at the sides and base of your skull.

Because most TMJ disorders are related to your head, neck, and shoulder muscles, practicing the following Deep Breathing, Relax Your Jaw, Stretch Your Jaw stretches, and the neck and shoulder stretches should provide you with instant relief. You'll find additional stretches to address TMJD in Chapter 3's "Upper Back, Shoulders, and Chest" section and Chapter 5's Receiving Stretch, Gentle Side Stretch, Gentle Twist, and Shoulder and Chest Expander stretches.

## Deep Breathing

Breathing deeply reduces stress, a major cause of TMJD. Because stress is part of daily living, it's important to practice Deep Breathing to enlist its support throughout the day. You'll release toxins, strengthen your lungs and diaphragm, massage your internal organs, and improve your ability to focus and think clearly.

1. Lie on your back on a firm yet comfortable surface, with your legs extended and your arms at your sides.

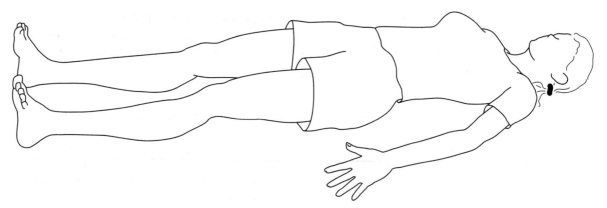

Lie on your back with your legs extended and your arms to your sides.

2. Place one hand on your chest and the other on your abdomen. Inhale deeply through your nostrils, feeling your lower hand rise as your belly expands. Your upper hand should move only slightly.

3. Exhale long and slowly through your nose, and then switch halfway through to exhaling through your mouth.

4. Practice breathing in this manner for eight deep breaths, focusing your attention on making the hand on your abdomen rise as much as you can.

## Relax Your Jaw

Relax Your Jaw is a vital exercise to manage TMJD. Relaxing your jaw allows it to stretch rather than remain in a constant contracted state. This stretch trains you to keep your jaw in a relaxed position all the time, allowing all the muscles that surround it to rest. Make it a part of your everyday routine.

1. Bring the tip of your tongue to the roof of your mouth behind, but not touching, your two front teeth. Keep your lips together, teeth slightly apart. Keep your lower jaw completely relaxed.

2. Take four breaths as deeply as you can without straining.

**A Stretch in Time ...**

Try stopping for a moment before you pick up the phone to practice Relax Your Jaw.

## Stretch Your Jaw

Stretch the muscles that close your jaw and loosen up those that open it. Make Stretch Your Jaw part of your daily routine by practicing it before you brush your teeth in the morning and at night.

**Flex Alert!**

If your jaw is sore, use moist heat over the affected area as you stretch. Avoid this stretch entirely if your jaw is extremely strained or you suffer from jaw popping or clicking.

1. Bring a hand up to your mouth and place the largest knuckle of your index finger between your teeth, resting your teeth and jaw there for eight long breaths. Close your eyes if you are steady, and consciously relax all your facial, neck, and shoulder muscles. Rest your arm for three breaths and notice how your jaw feels.

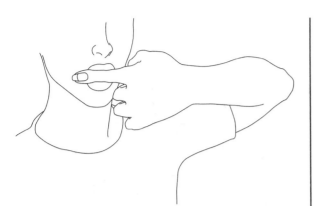

**Place the knuckle of your index finger between your teeth.**

2. Continue with step 1, but this time place two knuckles and then three knuckles between your teeth. When you are finished, rest your arm and jaw for four deep breaths and notice how your mouth and jaw feel.

### S-t-r-e-t-c-h It Out

Be careful not to create tension in your face, neck, shoulders, or arms as you practice Stretch Your Jaw. Deliberately loosen your muscles by taking long, deep breaths, concentrating on your exhale as you stretch.

# Nursing Your Neck

Perhaps you suffer from chronic tension, pain, and discomfort in your neck. If so, you're not alone. Your head weighs about 10 pounds—holding that up all day places a constant strain on your neck muscles. Your head may feel lighter if you stretch.

As you move through your stretching routine, keep your neck aligned with the rest of your spine. Allow your neck to naturally bend forward and gently bend backward. Never let your head drop back too deeply or roll your head around on your neck, as head-rolling exercises don't respect the structure of the vertebrae in your neck.

### Flex Alert!

If you have a neck condition such as arthritis, neck pain, or numbness; spurs on your cervical vertebrae; or herniated cervical intervertebral discs, practice the following stretches cautiously. If you feel pain or your condition worsens, back off and consult your physician.

The neck stretches that follow serve to gently stretch and loosen neck muscles. Always move gradually, gliding your head and neck into position.

## Seated Neck Stretch

Give the small muscles of your neck a rest as you stretch and lengthen them, improving your posture and increasing circulation simultaneously. If you suffer from neck injury or pain, stretch with care, especially if your pain increases or you feel numbness.

1. Sit on a chair with a firm seat, your spine straight. Take three long breaths, feeling the length of your spinal column as you breathe. With your chin parallel to the floor, let go of any tension you may be holding in your jaw, neck, and shoulders with every exhale.

2. Inhale deeply and gently lift your head toward the sky. As you exhale, slowly allow your head to move sideways and your right ear to move toward your right shoulder. Keep your eyes open and look down, keeping your jaw relaxed. *Do not raise your shoulder toward your ear or lift your chin.* Hold this passive stretch for four breaths.

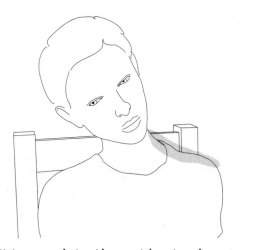

**Sitting on a chair with a straight spine, drop your right ear to your right shoulder, your eyes open and looking down.**

3. Repeat step 2, this time allowing your left ear to move toward your left shoulder. Practice two more sets.

### A Stretch in Time ...

Save time and stretch your neck and jaw by combining Relax Your Jaw with the Seated Neck Stretch.

## Kneeling Neck Stretch

If you suffer from chronic tension in your neck and shoulders or tightness or pain between your shoulder blades, you can find relief with the Kneeling Neck Stretch. You'll strengthen and gently stretch your neck as you loosen tight hips and stretch your lower back.

1. On a mat or blanket, sit on your heels and rest your hands on your thighs. Notice where you feel a stretch.

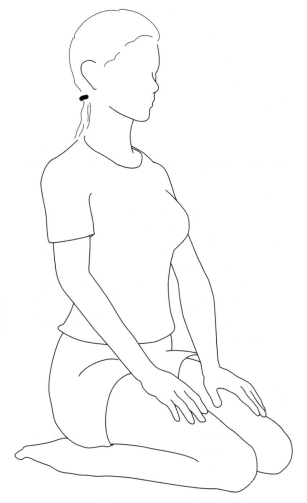

**Sitting on your heels, rest your hands on your thighs.**

2. Gaze straight ahead. Inhale and sweep your left arm wide and up by your left ear, making a half-circle, as you lift your hips up off your heels.

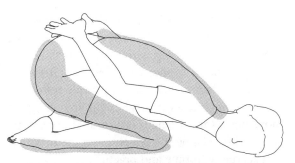

Fold forward on your knees, resting the back of your hands on your lower back. Turn your head to the right, placing your left cheek on the floor.

4. Inhale and lift your hips off your heels, sweeping your right arm wide and up by your right ear. Let the back of your left hand remain on your lower back.

5. As you exhale, bend forward, sweeping your right arm behind your back, bringing the back of your right hand to your lower back to meet your left hand. Turn your head slowly to the left, resting the right side of your head on the floor.

6. Repeat steps 2 through 5 three more times, ending by sitting on your heels and resting with your hands on your thighs.

# Stretching Sore Shoulders

Your neck and shoulders are connected, so it makes sense that neck and shoulder pain are often interrelated. Driving, constantly reaching or pushing, using poor posture, playing sports, and carrying heavy objects may exacerbate shoulder discomfort and pain.

If you were told to "hold your shoulders up" as a child, by now, as an adult, your shoulder and neck muscles have been shaped by years of holding your body in an incorrect posture. When you expand your chest as you stretch, you'll breathe fully and develop a greater freedom of movement, returning your shoulders to a more normal alignment.

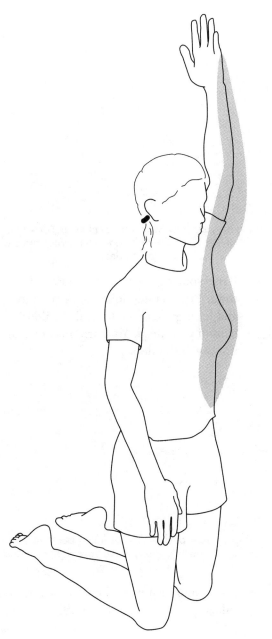

Standing on your knees, sweep your left arm up while rotating your palm in.

3. As you exhale, bend forward, sweeping your left arm behind your back, bringing the backs of your hands to your lower back. Turn your head slowly to the right, resting the left side of your head on the floor.

If you suffer from *frozen shoulder*, your range of movement is markedly decreased. In this case, restrict your stretching within a comfortable range of motion. Upper-back stretches, massage, warm baths, and rest can provide relief. As your condition improves, so might your range of movement. Improvement occurs after consistent care and stretching. Be patient, and the benefits will accrue with time and practice.

**Flexicon** _____

**Frozen shoulder,** or *adhesive capsulitis,* is a condition in which the shoulder capsule, the connective tissue surrounding your shoulder joint, becomes irritated and inflexible, causing severe loss of mobility in your shoulder.

## Supine Shoulder Stretch

The next time you're not up to par or are feeling tired and need a stress-free way to unwind, nurture your shoulders with the Supine Shoulder Stretch. These delicious movements expand your chest, soothe aching shoulders, and calm your mind. This routine is a perfect way to end your day as you prepare for a good night's rest. The asymmetrical movements allow you to examine each shoulder and notice any differences between them. A side benefit is the way the stretch allows you to relax your back and stretch in a comfortable manner.

1. Lie on your back, your knees bent, your feet on the floor even with your hips and parallel, your arms at your sides. Close your eyes, take a few breaths, and let all your muscles relax.

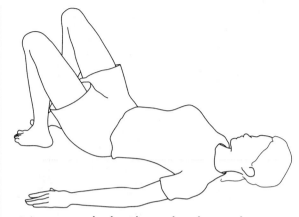

Lying on your back with your bent knees, place your feet on the floor hip-width apart with your arms at your sides.

2. Raise your right arm over your head toward the ceiling, inhaling as you move, and let it glide down toward the floor behind your head. Your arm may or may not touch the floor.

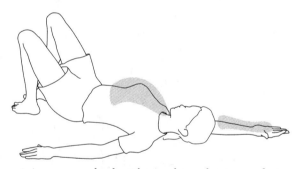

Lying on your back with your knees bent, your feet on floor hip-width apart, move your right arm back over your head.

3. Move your arm up and back down by your side as you exhale, ending in the starting position.

4. Repeat steps 2 and 3, increasing the stretch so your arm moves farther down toward the floor behind your head, three more times on each side, alternating arms.

## Sun and Earth

Address chronic shoulder and neck tension or pain as well as recurring headaches with the Sun and Earth stretch. These simple movements of your arms and shoulders, coordinated with breathing, expand your chest and increase mobility in your upper back, neck, and shoulders. It may help you rest easier, too.

1. On a mat or blanket, sit on your heels, rest your hands on your thighs, and notice where you feel a stretch.

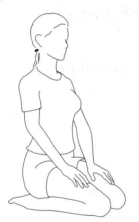

Sitting on your heels, rest your hands on your thighs.

2. Inhaling, sweep your arms wide, making a big circle, as you lift your hips off your heels. Stretch your arms over your head and bring your palms together. You may keep your arms shoulder-width apart if your shoulders are tight.

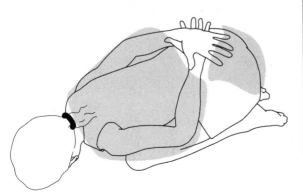

Standing on your knees, stretch your arms over your head, bringing your palms together.

3. As you exhale, bend forward, sweeping your arms wide, with the backs of your hands landing on your lower back and your palms turned upward.

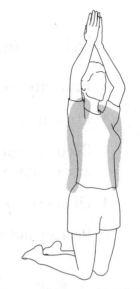

Forward fold on your knees. Place the backs of your hands on your sacrum with your palms turned up.

4. Inhale, lift your hips off your heels, and continue moving through steps 2 and 3 four more times.

5. End as you sit on your heels and rest with your hands on your thighs.

## The Least You Need to Know

◆ Find relief from headaches by stretching as soon as you feel pain, positioning your head below your heart.

◆ Keeping the tip of your tongue at the roof of your mouth behind your two front teeth helps relieve a tight jaw.

◆ It might feel great to roll your head around your neck, but doing so could damage the vertebrae in your neck.

◆ Time, patience, and diligent stretching of your chest and shoulders bring your shoulders into normal alignment.

# In This Chapter

◆ Elasticity = the end of joint pain and stiffness

◆ Prevent and treat carpal tunnel syndrome

◆ Become supple and strong with four fun ways to move your body

◆ Discover how good it feels to loosen your hips

◆ Protect and nurture your knees

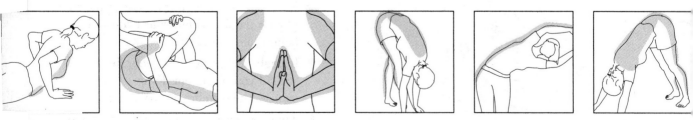

# Chapter 7

# Easing Joint Pain and Stiffness

Your joints shoulder a heavy burden, supporting your muscles and bones. Years of stress and strain, as well as previous injuries, can leave joints more susceptible to pain and stiffness. Aging is a major cause of joint pain and stiffness, but you don't have to accept it! Nor do you have to believe that medication is your only hope for relief.

It's important to take care of your hips and knees, the two largest and most important and vulnerable joints in your body. Stretching the muscles that support these joints is a great alternative to jarring, high-impact aerobic exercise that can cause hip and knee pain and injury. With the stretches in this chapter, you strengthen and stretch the muscles and connective tissue that support your hips and knees—a natural method to prevent and relieve pain.

Other routines focus on your other critical joints, such your hands and wrists, to prevent and treat carpal tunnel syndrome. You learn how to position your body to relieve pressure on your joints and to restore mobility lost because of arthritis and *osteoarthritis*. You also practice proper sitting and standing posture to support your joints throughout all your daily activities. When your joints feel tight, sore, and tired after a long day, you'll discover how stretching is a delicious way to unwind. Or if you want to warm up, you'll be able to practice gentle stretches before moving on to more intense exercises.

Beyond the routines themselves, you'll find out when to practice certain stretches and how to breathe to support your muscles and joints. While you stretch, you'll be directed to observe the differences in sensations between your right and left knees, hips, arms, and legs. In some routines, you'll have fun using props to comfortably support your muscles, bones, and joints as you safely stretch to keep yourself flexible and pain-free.

# Carpal Tunnel Syndrome

Carpal tunnel syndrome (CTS) is a condition that arises when the median nerve, which runs from your forearm into your hand, becomes pressed or squeezed at the wrist, causing pain, numbness, coldness, and weakness in parts of the hand. Symptoms may gradually increase over time, and repetitive activities, physiology, and family history play major roles in the development of CTS.

If you suffer from CTS, the idea of stretching your sore wrists might seem absurd. But many stretching experts say that stretching may offer just the healing you need and that specific stretches may assist in wrist renewal. Movements that stretch out the upper back, neck, shoulders, arms, hands, and wrists can counteract the repetitive movements that cause CTS and may help prevent and treat the condition.

In addition to the specific stretches offered in Chapter 7, the following stretches from Chapter 3 can help prevent and treat CTS:

◆ Figure Eight

◆ Relaxing Chest Opener

◆ Chest Expander

◆ Prayer

◆ Finger Wrap

◆ Wrist Waves

◆ Wrist Circles

These stretches in Chapter 5 address CTS, too:

◆ Receiving Stretch

◆ Gentle Side Stretch

◆ Gentle Twist

◆ Shoulder and Chest Expander

◆ Strong Side Stretch

◆ Strong Twist

# Entire Front Stretch

With these simple movements, you stretch the front of your body from your hips through your belly, ribs, chest, shoulders, arms, and hands, all the way to your fingertips. You also stimulate spinal nerves by moving your arms forward and up by your ears. This stretch is a great warm-up to the stretches that follow, too.

1. Stand with your feet parallel and even with your hips. Rest your arms beside your body. Tuck your chin. Inhale, and relax as you exhale with your knees slightly bent.

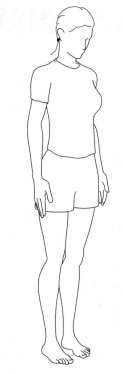

Stand with your feet parallel and hip-width apart. Place your arms beside your body with your chin tucked.

2. S-t-r-e-t-c-h your arms forward and up by your ears as you inhale. Gradually spread your fingers wide, palms facing forward. Feel the entire front of your body, chest, arms, hands, and fingers s-t-r-e-t-c-h.

## Pretzel

Perhaps you remember Pretzel from the "Upper Back, Shoulders, and Chest" section in Chapter 3. It's also perfect for preventing and treating CTS, as it stretches your upper back, neck, shoulders, elbows, forearms, wrists, hands, and fingers.

**Flex Alert!** _____

Stop stretching if you feel pain, and consult your physician.

1. Sit in a sturdy chair on a firm seat with a straight spine. Keep your jaw loose, your shoulders relaxed, and your chin parallel to the floor. Straighten both arms in front of your torso at shoulder level, with your palms skyward. Bend your right elbow and place it in the crease of your left elbow.

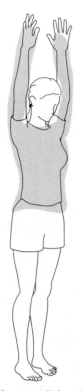

Stand with your feet parallel and hip-width apart. Stretch your arms all the way up, your palms facing forward with your fingers spread wide, your chin tucked.

3. S-t-r-e-t-c-h your arms forward and back down to your sides, relaxing your arms, palms, and fingers as you exhale.

4. Repeat steps 2 and 3 three additional times. As you repeat the movement, intensify the stretch as you press your arms back past your ears and open your fingers wide. Reach through your fingertips. Be careful to keep your elbows straight. Relax and observe the aftereffects.

**A Stretch in Time ...** _____

Start your day off with the Entire Front Stretch. Adding this one stretch to your morning routine wakes you up, gets your blood flowing, and expands your chest so you can breathe more easily all day long.

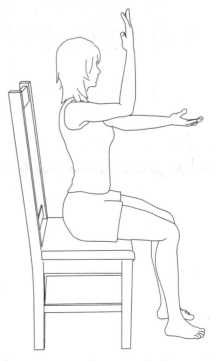

Sit with your arms out from your shoulders and place your right elbow in the crease of your left elbow.

2. Entwine your arms until you can place the fingers of your left hand on your right palm. If you can't touch your fingers to your palm, bring them to your wrist or forearm in a loose wrap.

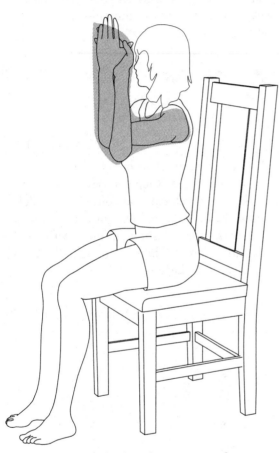

Sit with a straight back and entwine your forearms.

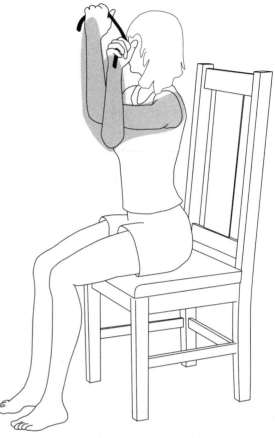

Sitting with your forearms entwined, hold a strap held in your left hand and grasp the other end with your right hand.

3. Move your elbows up or down slowly, and hold the stretch for four deep breaths, sitting steadily. Each time you inhale, imagine your upper back expanding. Picture your upper-back muscles becoming soft and pliable as you exhale. You may close your eyes to notice where you feel the stretch in your body.

4. Release your arms, let your hands rest on your thighs, and observe the difference in how your shoulders feel.

5. Repeat steps 1 through 4, placing your left elbow in the crease of your right elbow, and once again hold your position for four breaths, noticing any variations as you stretch this side.

# Reclining Fork

Reclining Fork covers all the bases for prevention and cure of carpal tunnel syndrome. No pressure is placed on your hands. You'll strengthen your back and shoulders to provide support to your head, neck, and chest; stretch and strengthen your abdominal muscles while you expand your chest; and strengthen your lungs and breathe more deeply to relieve stress.

1. Lie on your belly, your forehead touching the floor, and place your palms flat on the floor, under your shoulders. Roll your shoulders up toward your ears and down the back of your body, with your shoulder blades together and your elbows hugging your body. Press the tops of your feet and your pubic bone into the floor.

2. As you inhale, slowly lift your chest off the floor, using your back muscles rather than your hands.

3. Lower your chest as you exhale. Lift your chest again as you inhale, and lower your chest as you exhale. Repeat these movements two more times, and then hold the stretch with your chest lifted off the floor for four breaths. Remember not to place any weight in your hands.

4. Release the stretch as you exhale. Rest and notice the results.

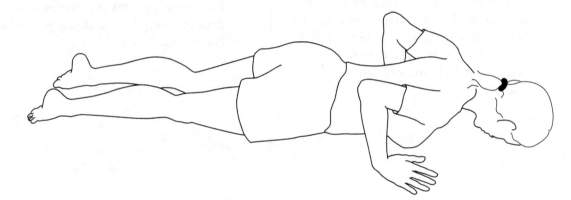

Lying on your belly, your forehead touching the floor, place your palms flat on the floor under your shoulders, your elbows hugging your body.

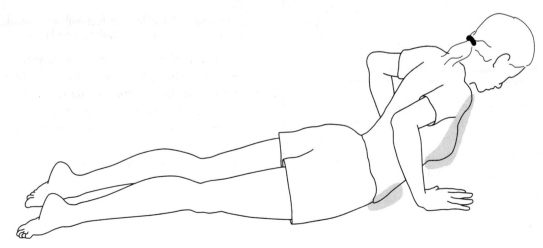

Lying on your belly with your palms flat on the floor under your shoulders, lift your chest.

# Bowl

This final stretch in the series of CTS stretches uses your body's leverage to stretch the entire front of your body, fingers, wrists, and hands.

**Flex Alert!** _____

The Reclining Fork and Bowl stretches might aggravate sore backs. If you feel tightness or pain in your lower back, omit these stretches from your routine. Omit Bowl from your routine if you suffer from back injury or inflammation, knee pain, high blood pressure, or a heart condition.

1. Lie on your belly, with your forehead and arms on the floor and your arms extended forward. Reach and stretch through your fingers and toes as if you're trying to touch the walls in front of you and behind you.

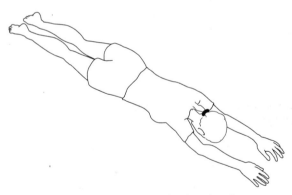

Lying on your belly with your forehead and arms on the floor, extend your arms forward.

2. Bend your knees, bringing your heels toward your hips. Reach your hands back, one at a time, and grasp the tops of your feet. Inhale deeply, and as you exhale, press your lower abdomen, pubic bone, and hips into the floor.

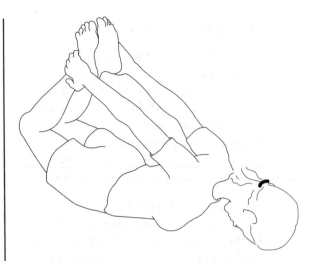

Lying on your belly with your forehead on the floor, grasp your feet ... and don't forget to breathe.

3. Press your feet into your hands as you draw in a deep breath, lifting your head, chest, shoulders, and knees.

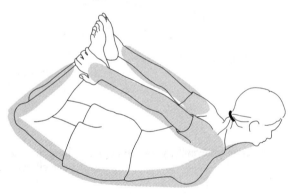

Lying on your belly, hold your feet with your hands. Keep your head, chest, shoulders, and knees up.

4. Return to the starting position as you exhale. Repeat the movements three more times, inhaling as you lift the front of your body and knees, exhaling as you lower your head, chest, and knees. Lift and hold the stretch for four breaths. Lower your head, chest, and knees as you exhale.

# Hip and Knee Remedies

Your knees and hips have much in common. These solid, dense, complex structures support nearly the entire weight of your body. Your knees and hips typically lose their range of motion over the course of a long-term sedentary lifestyle, so stretching is a highly effective way to restore their mobility. Hips and knees are also vulnerable to injury and *osteoarthritis*. It's wise, therefore, to take the time to strengthen and stabilize the muscles and connective tissue that support these essential joints.

> **Flexicon**
>
> **Osteoarthritis** is a condition in which joints become inflamed and painful, caused by the degeneration of the cartilage that protects and acts as a cushion inside your joints. Osteoarthritis affects nearly 21 million people in the United States.

All hip and knee stretches are gentle in contrast to jarring, high-impact aerobic exercise that may result in hip and knee pain and injury. You perform these stretches lying on your back with your legs elevated to relieve joint pressure. You can practice these stretches when your hips and knees feel tight and sore, or when you're tired after a long day.

> **S-t-r-e-t-c-h It Out**
>
> Always practice the Single Knee Bends, Reclining Hip Flexor Stretch, or Triangle Stretch after the Reclining Fork and Bowl stretches (earlier in this chapter), to release any accumulated tension and stretch your back.

## Single Knee Bends

Single Knee Bends alleviate knee joint discomfort as you stretch and strengthen the muscles that support your knees. This reclining stretch takes pressure off your hips and knees by stretching your hamstrings, your calves, and the soles of your feet. Also an asymmetric stretch, it allows you to investigate the differences between your right and left sides.

1. Lie on your back, your chin toward your chest, your knees bent, your left foot on the floor, your right foot lifted, and your right thigh toward your chest, with your hands clasped in the crook of your right knee. Bend your right knee and elbows.

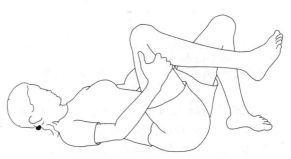

Lying on your back, your chin toward your chest, your left foot on the floor and your right foot lifted, clasp your right thigh toward your chest while bending your right knee and your elbows.

2. Slowly straighten your right leg, stretching your foot toward the ceiling as you inhale, with your arms straight. Flex your right foot, but keep your right knee slightly bent. Keep your chin down toward your chest.

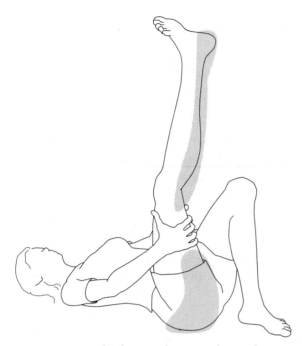

Lying on your back, your chin toward your chest, your left foot on the floor, and your right leg straight. Slightly bend your right knee, with your right foot flexed.

3. Exhale as you bend your right knee back to your starting position.

4. Repeat steps 2 and 3 five more times. Then practice the Single Knee Bend six times with your left leg. Rest with your feet on the floor, your knees bent, and your arms at your sides.

## Reclining Hip Flexor Stretch

The Reclining Hip Flexor Stretch stimulates your digestive system and increases flexibility in your lower back, hips, and legs. Practicing this relaxing stretch one side at a time affords you the opportunity to notice any differences in your right and left hips.

**Flex Alert!** _____

Do not practice this stretch after the third month of pregnancy or if you've had recent abdominal surgery.

1. Lie on your back with your legs out-stretched and your arms beside your body. Inhale deeply, and as you exhale, bend your right knee toward your chest and interlace your fingers below your right knee, gently holding your right thigh toward your chest. Do not force or pull your leg.

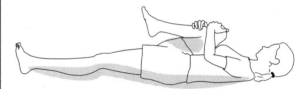

Lying on your back, with your left leg outstretched and your right knee toward your chest, interlace your fingers below your right knee.

2. Hold the stretch for four long, smooth, deep breaths. Keep your shoulders and jaw relaxed. Straighten your right leg very slowly as you inhale to release the stretch. Pause to take a few breaths, noticing both sides of your body.

3. Practice the stretch on the left side by repeating steps 1 and 2, drawing your left thigh toward your chest.

# Triangle Stretch

Create a triangle shape using your arms and legs, and watch your lower back and hips relax. Although the Triangle Stretch may produce intense sensations, once you unwind, you'll feel a release of tension. A perfect stretch for those suffering from a sore or tight lower back, this stretch allows you to examine each hip and side of your back in isolation.

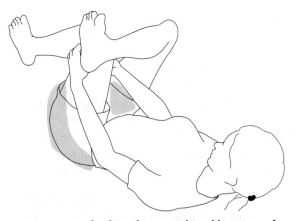

Lying on your back, with your right ankle on top of your left thigh below your knee, clasp your hands under your left thigh, with your fingers interlaced and your chin toward your chest.

### Flex Alert!

Proceed with caution if you suffer from knee pain or inflammation or if you have recently had knee surgery. If you experience pain as you move into the Triangle Stretch, back off! Perhaps you can try it again when your knees aren't as tender.

1. Lie on your back, with your arms beside your body, your feet flat on the floor, and your knees bent. Take a few deep breaths to relax your muscles.

2. Pick up your right foot, placing your right ankle on top of your left thigh below your knee, as if you are crossing your legs. Reach with your right hand through the triangle you've formed with your legs, and bring your left hand under your left thigh, interlacing your fingers. Keep your chin toward your chest. If your neck feels strained, place a pillow under your head. Be as comfortable as you can while you hold this position for four long deep breaths.

3. Unwrap your legs and return to your starting position, outlined in step 1. Take a few breaths and notice how your hips and back feel and whether you experience any difference between the two sides.

4. Pick up your left foot, placing your left ankle on top of your right thigh below the knee, as if you are crossing your legs. Reach with your left hand through the triangle you've formed with your legs, and bring your right hand under your right thigh, interlacing your fingers. Keep your chin toward your chest. Hold the stretch for four deep breaths.

5. Return to your starting position, taking a few relaxing breaths.

### S-t-r-e-t-c-h It Out

If you cannot clasp your hands under your thigh, use a strap. Place the strap under your thigh and hold the ends of the strap with your hands.

## Outer Thigh Stretch

The Outer Thigh Stretch is a wonderful addition to your stretching routine, as it addresses hip, hamstring, lower-back, and abdominal concerns. It strengthens the musculature of your hips and abdominal muscles, increases the flexibility of your spine, and stimulates your spinal nerves. You'll also release stress and feel rejuvenated after performing this powerful stretch.

1. Lie on your back, with your legs straight and your arms out in a *T*.

2. As you exhale, lift your left leg toward the sky at a 90-degree angle from your torso. As you inhale, stretch up through your left heel.

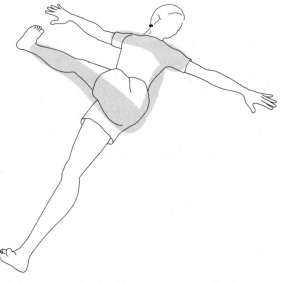

Lying on your back with your arms stretched to a T, move your left leg to the floor by your right hand and turn your head to the left.

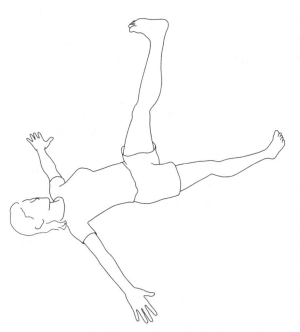

Lying on your back, your arms stretched out in a T, lift your left leg to a 90-degree angle.

3. Exhale and bring your left foot to the floor toward your right hand as you turn your head slowly to the left.

4. Inhale and move your left leg toward the sky, keeping your left foot flexed.

5. Repeat steps 3 and 4 three more times, breathing as you move.

6. Hold the stretch for four breaths, keeping your left foot off the floor. Keep your neck as relaxed as possible. You can support your left leg with a strap, if needed.

7. To release the stretch, inhale as you lift your left leg, exhale as you hold your leg up, and inhale again as you lower your left leg to meet your right leg. Exhale and rest for a moment.

8. Repeat steps 1 through 7, moving the right leg this time. Relax on your back and feel the effects of the stretch.

**A Stretch in Time ...**

The stretches in the "Hip and Knee Remedies" section are perfect for calming frazzled nerves at the end of the day. They're all practiced on your back so you don't need a lot of energy. You can even move into these positions as you watch television.

## The Least You Need to Know

◆ Exercising is painful for those suffering from joint pain and stiffness. Stretching after a good warm-up is a beneficial alternative.

◆ Don't wait for symptoms of carpal tunnel syndrome to appear. Practicing the carpal tunnel stretches is your best insurance.

◆ Loosening your hips can relieve pain in your hips and lower back, as well as restore lost mobility.

◆ Stretching is a perfect alternative to high-impact aerobic activity that can cause or aggravate knee issues.

# In This Chapter

◆ Basic techniques to prevent and treat back pain

◆ Six simple methods guaranteed to relax your back

◆ Prevent and treat sciatica now

◆ Strengthen your back without strain

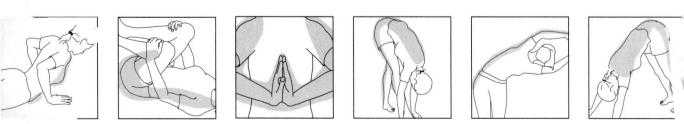

# Chapter 8

# Sore Backs Stop Here

A host of common culprits cause lower back pain. You might have sciatica, a debilitating and widespread condition caused by irritation of the sciatic nerve characterized by shooting pain down the back of your leg. Perhaps you have a flattened curve in your lower back or tight hamstrings. Maybe your abdominal muscles or back muscles are weak.

Whatever the source of pain, because backaches frequently result from a battle between your abdominal muscles and your hamstrings, you risk causing difficulties if you haphazardly target these areas. Exercising to strengthen your abdominal muscles can inadvertently aggravate your sore back or increase tension in your neck and shoulders. Often the very steps that comprise a good back care program may actually hurt your back if they're not practiced properly or in the correct sequence.

A carefully constructed stretching routine is an important first step in learning how to safely care for your back. Therefore, in this chapter, you learn how to properly strengthen and relax your back, prevent and treat sciatica, and use simple methods to treat your sore back. You'll become skilled at following proper alignment and movement patterns that protect your back from injury and aggravation.

As you practice safe stretches, postures, specific techniques, and self-care strategies, you'll accomplish important back care goals, such as strengthening your abdominal muscles, stretching your hamstrings, and strengthening your back muscles. You'll also get good advice on what to do when back pain strikes, explore breathing techniques that naturally stretch your spine, and arm yourself with observational skills you can employ to support the natural structure of your spine.

Most important, have some fun when you stretch. Support your back with easy-to-find props. Feel free to modify the routines to make them more comfortable. Practice stretches to address your particular health concerns. Your back supports you. Isn't it time to give some support back?

# Essential Ways to Treat a Sore Back

If you've strained your back or are experiencing continual soreness, try these methods to find relief:

◆ Lie on your back with a bolster (a long, narrow pillow or cushion) under your knees and relax.

◆ Lie on your side, hug a pillow, and drape your leg over the pillow.

◆ Sit with a straight spine, getting up to stretch every 30 minutes.

◆ Take a hot Epsom salt bath at least once a day.

◆ Apply heat to the painful area to loosen contracted muscles.

### S-t-r-e-t-c-h It Out

Don't forget to warm up before you stretch, and always use envelope breathing.

Once you feel ready to move, a regular stretching program is your best insurance to avoid enduring life with a sore back. Although you may have the best intentions, perhaps you've learned the hard way that exercise doesn't suit you or that the tasks of daily living generate or aggravate back pain. The following stretches are specifically designed to prevent soreness and treat your aching back.

### Flex Alert!

Always obtain a thorough evaluation of your condition and advice about exercises with a qualified health-care professional before starting any exercise program. Consult your health-care adviser if you experience worsening of your pain, persistent pain even when lying down, or weakness or numbness in your legs or arms after practicing any of the following stretches.

## Relax Your Back on the Ball

Although lying on a ball might sound silly, it actually does relax your back. The ball works to elevate your spine and back muscles, allowing you to use the force of gravity to relax your back. Normally, your back supports your body while you sit or stand, or is pressed against a flat surface while you sleep. By lifting your back off the floor in a reclining position and using the ball to support your back, you can fully relax your back muscles without a bed or floor impeding them.

### S-t-r-e-t-c-h It Out

For this stretch, you need a 5-inch playground ball, available at from most sporting goods stores.

1. Gather your ball and find a quiet place where you can lie down on a firm surface. Choose a carpet or blanket, not a bed or couch. Lie on your side, roll onto your back, bend your knees, and place the soles of your feet hip-width apart. Place the ball within reach, rest your arms by your sides, and inhale deeply. As you exhale, consciously release tension from your whole body.

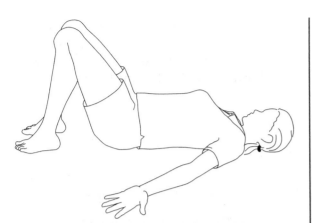

Lying on your back with your feet hip-width apart and parallel, place your arms beside your body.

2. Holding the ball in one hand, lift your hips just high enough to place the ball under your *sacrum*. With your palms facing up, place your arms at a 45-degree angle away from your torso. If you feel unsteady, move your arms directly by your sides, palms down to stabilize your torso. Remain in this position for eight long, deep breaths, letting go of tension with every exhale.

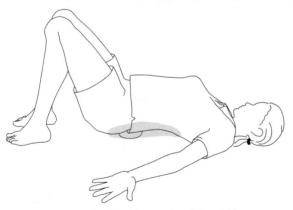

Lying on your back with your feet hip-width apart and parallel, place your arms at a 45-degree angle away from your torso with your palms up and a 5-inch playground ball under your sacrum.

## Arch and Curl

How often do you allow yourself to do nothing except breathe as deeply as you can? This routine harnesses the power of your breath to naturally stretch your spine. Deep breathing coupled with a relaxed body enables you to create space between the vertebrae in your spine without exerting any effort.

1. Lie on your back. Keep your feet parallel and even with your hips, and place your arms away from your torso at a 45-degree angle, your palms up. This starting position is the same for Relax Your Back on the Ball (except without the ball).

2. Inhale deeply into your chest, and exhale slowly to release bodily tension. As you continue to breathe into your chest as deeply as you can, feel your upper back arch off the floor. Then, without tensing your legs or arms, engage your abdominal muscles and exhale all your breath out.

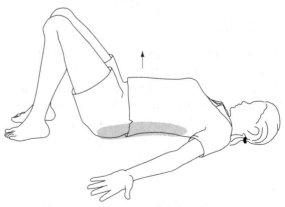

Lying on your back, your feet hip-width apart and parallel, your arms at a 45-degree angle away from your torso with your palms up, arch your upper back off the floor.

3. Once you create a long, deep, rhythmic breathing cycle, begin to add a pause for a few seconds at the top of each inhale and the bottom of each exhale. Continue breathing this way, concentrating on your breath. Continue to feel your upper back and spine arching at the top of the inhale, and your lower back and tailbone curling toward your nose at the bottom of the exhale. Practice eight breaths this way and then pause to notice the effects of the natural stretch.

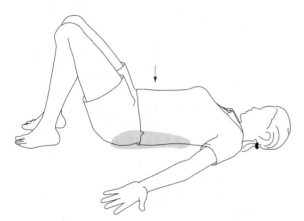

Lying on your back, your feet hip-width apart and parallel, your arms at a 45-degree angle away from your torso with your palms up, lower your back and tailbone and curl toward your nose.

## Knee Press

The Knee Press is such an essential part of your stretching program that you'll see it again in Chapters 9 and 11. This reclining stretch is the perfect way to respond when back soreness strikes. It's also the best preventive medicine, for in addition to stretching your back and hips, this stretch helps strengthen your abdominal muscles and calm your busy mind.

1. Lie on your back on a comfortable surface (but not your bed). Inhale deeply. As you exhale, draw one knee toward your chest. Inhale again, and with the next exhale, draw your other knee toward your chest. Place your hands lightly on each knee. Tuck your chin toward your chest while keeping your head on the floor.

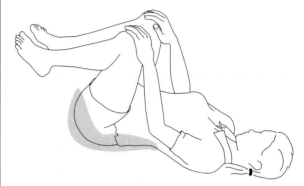

Lying on your back, bend your knees toward your chest, with one hand on each knee and your elbows bent.

2. Move your thighs away from your chest as you inhale and straighten your arms. Keep your hands on your knees. Move your thighs toward your chest, bending your elbows as you exhale. Do not pull or force your legs toward your chest. Practice these movements eight times.

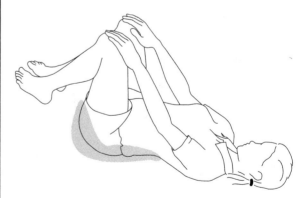

Lying on your back with your knees bent, rest one hand on each knee and extended and straighten your arms.

### Flex Alert! _____

Step 3 of the Knee Press requires much more exertion than steps 1 and 2. Do not practice step 3 if you have had recent abdominal surgery or if you experience pain after trying one repetition.

3. With your head resting on the floor, grasp your arms around your knees to form your body into a ball. Hold on to your hand, wrist, or forearm as you draw your knees toward your chest. Rest your head on the floor. Take one deep, full breath in this position. Inhale, and as you exhale, bring your nose toward your knees, engaging your abdominal muscles as you move.

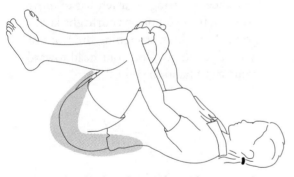

**Lying on your back with your knees bent, wrap your arms around your legs, keeping your head on the floor.**

4. Lower your upper back to the floor and relax your shoulders as you inhale. Repeat these movements two more times, then rest with your hands on your knees for a few moments.

## Z Stretch

The Z Stretch helps you become aware of your naturally curvy spine and rejuvenates your spinal column by keeping it supple. The flowing movements loosen your spine and release tension from your muscles, joints, and ligaments.

### S-t-r-e-t-c-h It Out _____

Use a firm, folded blanket under your knees to protect these precious parts of your body.

1. Kneel on a blanket or rug with your knees placed directly beneath your hips and your shoulders positioned directly above your wrists. Spread your fingers wide. Relax your shoulders. Inhale deeply into your chest, lifting your chin slightly at the top of the breath.

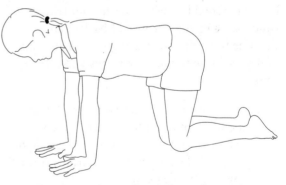

**Kneel with your knees directly beneath your hips, your shoulders positioned directly above your wrists and your fingers spread.**

2. As you exhale, bring your chin toward your chest, your chest toward your thighs, and your hips toward your heels, moving into a crouching position like the letter Z.

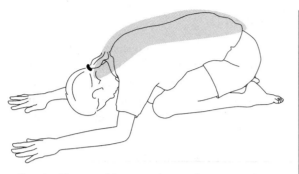

Kneel with your chin toward your chest, your chest toward your thighs, and your hips toward your heels.

3. Repeat steps 1 and 2 seven more times, and then rest in the Z position for four deep breaths.

## Knee as Handle

Now it's time to stretch your quadriceps muscles, located at the front of your thighs. Knee as Handle gently lengthens these muscles that may have tightened because of tense hamstrings, which are a common cause of back strain. Practice this safe and relaxing stretch any time of day as a way to relax your back and release stress.

1. Lie on your back with your feet flat and about a foot and a half apart. Place your arms away from your torso at an angle of about 45 degrees, with your palms turned upward. Inhale deeply.

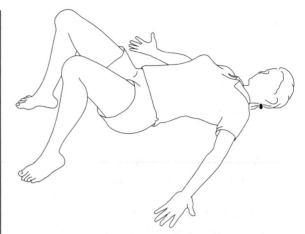

Lying on your back with your feet flat and about 1½ feet apart, move your arms about 45 degrees away from your torso, turn your palms upward, and breathe!

2. Move your right knee down toward your left knee, allowing your left leg to move to the left as you press your right knee toward the floor, stretching the front of your right thigh. Roll your head toward your right hand as you exhale.

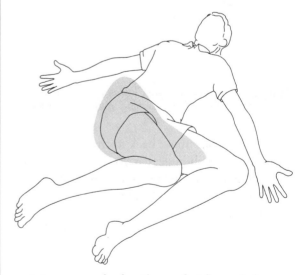

Lying on your back with your feet flat and about 1½ feet apart, move your arms about 45 degrees away from your torso, move your right knee down toward your left knee, move your left leg toward the left, and press your knee toward the floor.

3. Move back to the starting position as you inhale. Move your left knee down toward your right knee, allowing your right leg to move to the right as you press your left knee toward the floor, stretching the front of your left thigh. Roll your head toward the left hand as you exhale.

4. Repeat steps 2 and 3 two more times, and then hold the stretch on each side for four deep breaths.

## Heels Over Head Stretch

You may remember this stretch from Chapter 6. Aside from relieving your throbbing head, you can use the Heels Over Head Stretch as a surefire way to gently stretch tight hamstrings. Anyone can practice this stretch, and it's a great way to relax and unwind after a long day.

1. Lie on your right side, close to a wall, with your knees bent toward your chest. Scoot your hips so your feet and buttocks touch the wall.

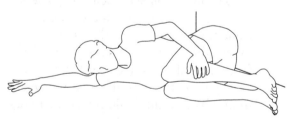

Lying on your right side with your knees bent, move so your feet and buttocks touch the wall.

2. Roll to the left, swinging your legs up the wall. Open your arms from your shoulders out to the sides, palms up. If you feel tension in the backs of your legs, turn your legs slightly in and release any tightness in your knees.

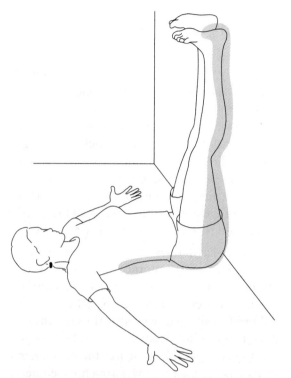

Lying on your back with your legs up the wall, stretch your arms out to your sides.

3. Relax into the stretch and breathe deeply, holding the position at least 5 minutes. Your breathing should become slow and deep as you hold the stretch, relieving stress and relaxing muscles in your forehead, eyes, jaw, and tongue.

4. Come out of the stretch retracing the steps you took to move into it. Bend your knees, roll to your side, and use your strong arms to move to your hands and knees. Place one foot on the floor, bend your knee, and hold on to a chair or the wall for support as you raise your body to standing.

### A Stretch in Time ...

It's important to practice back-relaxation stretches every day. Try rotating through the stretches in the "Essential Ways to Treat a Sore Back" section, practicing a different one each day.

# Dealing With Sciatica

As many as 1 million Americans suffer from sciatica, a condition characterized by pain in the buttocks and lower back. Other sensations—including severe pain, tingling, numbness, heat, and even sensations similar to an electric shock—may radiate down the back of the leg through the calf to the foot. Lasting anywhere from a few hours to several weeks, sciatica can start as an aching sensation that makes it hard to sit and eventually intensifies as an incapacitating pain that affects your ability to move.

Sciatica has various causes, the most common of which is a ruptured disc that encroaches on the root of the sciatic nerve. The condition commonly occurs when the soft gel-like material inside a spinal disc escapes through the disc's outer lining. Sciatica can also be caused by osteoarthritis, which injures the sciatic nerve by narrowing the opening through which nerve roots leave the lower spine. Yet another cause is Piriformis syndrome, which occurs when the *piriformis muscle* impinges on the sciatic nerve.

**Flexicon** _____

The **piriformis muscle** extends from the side of the sacrum to the top of the thigh bone at the hip joint, passing over the sciatic nerve.

An estimated 300,000 Americans a year resort to a variety of methods to alleviate the symptoms of sciatica: anti-inflammatory medications, acupressure, epidural injections, ice applications—even surgery. Significantly, a 2006 study published in *The Journal of the American Medical Association* found that those suffering from ruptured discs in their lower backs recover whether or not they have surgery. Given these findings, stretching and strengthening the back are essential therapies to speed the healing process and to seek relief from pain in the meantime. But results won't happen overnight—so patience and discipline are also prerequisites for managing your sciatica.

## Seated Sciatic Stretch

If a short, tight piriformis muscle is the cause of your sciatica, this stretch is for you. The Seated Sciatic Stretch gently stretches the piriformis if you practice it regularly. The key word is *gentle*, so be kind to yourself.

**S-t-r-e-t-c-h It Out** _____

You need to sit on at least one blanket for this stretch. You may need to add more blankets to increase the depth of the cushion.

1. Sit on a folded blanket. Bend your knees and place your feet flat on the floor in front of you. Move your right thigh toward the floor as you place your right foot on the floor beside your left hip. Now place your left foot on the floor near the front of your right thigh. If your foot does not reach the floor or the stretch is too intense, place your foot next to or in front of your right knee. Check to see that your weight rests evenly on both hips. Place additional blankets under your buttocks for support, if you need to.

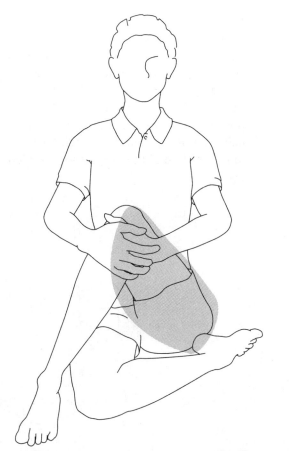

Sitting on a folded blanket with your right thigh toward the floor, your right foot on the floor beside your left hip, your left foot on the floor near the front of your right thigh, rest your hands on your left shin below your knee.

2. Draw in a deep breath as you lengthen your spine, lift the crown of your head toward the sky, and exhale. Place your hands below your left knee. You may move deeper into the stretch by bringing your left knee toward the right side of your chest.

3. Hold the stretch for six breaths to begin. As you practice the stretch, work up to holding your breath for several minutes. You may go deeper into the stretch by

placing your hands on the floor in front of you and leaning forward as you exhale.

4. Repeat the stretch on the other side, noticing whether the stretch feels different on this side. Practice two to four sets.

**Flex Alert!**

This stretch places your piriformis in a stretched position. If you have sciatic pain caused by a short piriformis, this stretch will exacerbate that pain. If you stretch too deeply, you may cause intense pain and perhaps even a muscle spasm. If you feel pain, adjust your position by increasing the height of the padding beneath you.

## One Leg Up, One Leg Down

This stretch is similar to the Heels Over Head Stretch. The only difference is that in One Leg Up, One Leg Down, you stretch one leg at a time, enabling you to notice the difference between your right and left legs. Practicing One Leg Up, One Leg Down releases your hamstrings and relieves sciatica as it gently stretches the entire back of your body. Using a doorframe to support your leg helps you relax as you reacquaint your legs and pelvis to their proper alignment.

1. Lie on your back next to a doorframe or post. Exhaling, lift your left leg and place it against the doorframe or post. Lengthen your right leg along the floor to position your legs at a 90-degree angle. Attempt to place your entire leg against the supporting surface. Bring your arms out from your body about 1 foot, with your palms turned up. Hold the stretch for four deep breaths while maintaining a relaxed body.

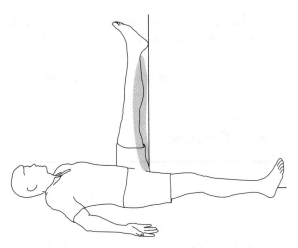

Lying on your back, with your left leg on a door-frame or post, stretch your right leg out along the floor and arms out from your body, your palms turned up.

2. Repeat the stretch with your right leg elevated.

### S-t-r-e-t-c-h It Out

When you first try One Leg Up, One Leg Down, you might not be able to rest your whole leg on the supporting surface. With continued practice and patience, though, you'll eventually move closer and closer to the 90-degree position.

## Reclining Right Angle

Those of you suffering from sciatica may safely stretch your elusive inner thigh muscles with the Reclining Right Angle stretch. This gentle stretch is similar to One Leg Up, One Leg Down, but you need a chair to support your leg, not a doorframe or post.

1. Find a chair and place it to your right. Lie on your back, positioning your body so you can rest your right leg out to the side on the chair.

2. Draw in a deep breath, and as you exhale, lift your right leg up toward the sky. Lengthen your leg as you inhale. Then, as you exhale, move your leg out to the right so the outside of your right foot rests on the chair. Keep your hips level and arms positioned out to your sides, with your palms up. Remain in the stretch for four long breaths and then repeat for your left leg.

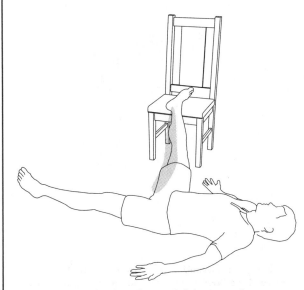

Lie on your back with your left leg straight, your right foot resting on a chair, your hips level, your arms out to the sides, and your palms turned up.

## Standing Right Angle

Conquer sciatica with this relaxing stretch. Carefully stretch your back with the aid of a table or countertop, bending your body forward halfway for support.

1. Facing a countertop or table, stand with your feet even with your hips. Your hip-bones should be level with the edge of the counter or table.

### S-t-r-e-t-c-h It Out

Stand on a block or step if you need to raise your hipbones to meet the edge of the table. If you're tall, place pillows or blankets on the tabletop where you're resting your torso so your body is positioned at a 90-degree angle.

2. With your arms outstretched, place your torso over the tabletop. Bend your elbows to reduce the intensity of the stretch, if you need to, or keep your arms straight to intensify the stretch. Your forehead should face the table. Allow your back to relax more deeply with each exhale. Hold the stretch for eight long breaths.

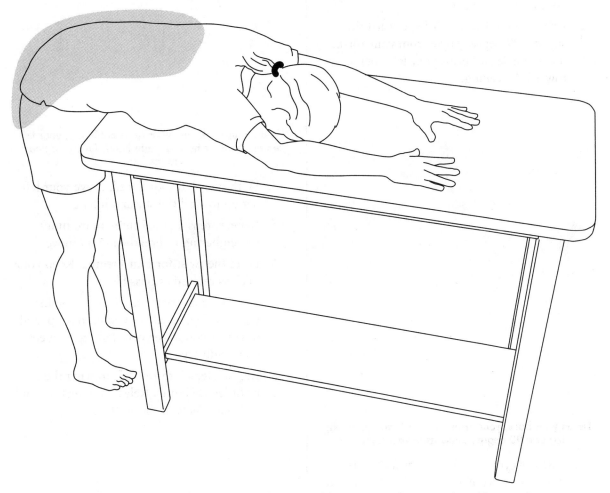

Stand with your feet hip-width apart, facing a table, your torso bent over the tabletop with your arms outstretched.

## Outer Thigh Stretch

Regularly practicing this stretch helps loosen tight outer-thigh muscles, a common cause of sciatica. It also increases the range of motion in your hips and groin. The prone position makes it safe for those with back issues.

1. Lie on your back, your legs straight and your arms out in a *T*.

2. Exhale and lift your left leg toward the sky at a 90-degree angle from your torso. Then inhale and press your left heel up toward the ceiling.

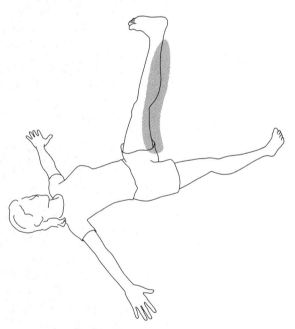

**Lie on your back, your arms out in a T, and your left leg at a 90-degree angle from your torso.**

3. Exhale as you bring your left foot to the floor toward your right hand and you turn your head slowly to the left.

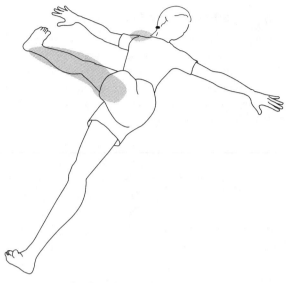

**Lie on your back with your arms out in a T, your left leg on the floor by your right hand. Turn your head to the left.**

4. With your left foot flexed, move your left leg up toward the sky and inhale.

5. Repeat steps 3 and 4 three more times, remembering to breathe as you move.

6. Hold the twist for four breaths. Keep your neck as relaxed as possible.

7. To release the stretch, inhale as you lift your left leg, exhale as you hold it up, and inhale as you lower your left leg to meet your right leg.

8. Repeat steps 1 through 7, moving the right leg this time. Relax on your back and feel the effects of the stretch.

# Back Strengtheners

You've made a wise decision to practice stretches that will result in a stronger back. However, if you suffer from back soreness, the idea of working your back muscles may seem intimidating.

Remember, though, that weak torso muscles attached to your spinal column may be the cause of your back strain. Strengthening your back muscles is effective because a stronger back helps you support your precious spine. The variety of stretches presented in this chapter helps you strengthen your back without strain.

### S-t-r-e-t-c-h It Out

Although in the past bed rest was often prescribed for severe back pain, the latest research indicates that a focused stretching and strengthening program is your best bet for managing back pain and your finest defense against its recurrence.

After you've practiced the back strengthening stretches, it's important to balance the work you've done by practicing a few stretches from the "Essential Ways to Treat a Sore Back" section of this chapter. In this manner, you'll relax the muscles you've just worked and release stress—a significant factor associated with the onset of back pain.

# Spinal Roll

A daily stretching routine is vital if you suffer from back soreness. Working in a stretch as part of your daily schedule is wise—it's just like brushing your teeth. The Spinal Roll is one of those stretches you can add with ease. It keeps your spine supple and gently strengthens your back muscles without strain. You can practice this stretch before you get out of bed in the morning or at bedtime.

1. Lie on your back, knees bent, feet placed a comfortable distance from your buttocks and hip-width apart. Rest your arms by your sides. Take a deep breath, and exhale as you roll your tailbone to your nose, flattening the natural curve at your lower back.

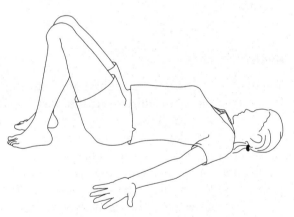

**Lying on your back with your knees bent, your feet hip-width apart, your arms by your sides, show no natural curve at your lower back.**

2. Inhale with your tailbone tucked, and slowly lift your hips as you exhale. With your hips lifted, take in a deep breath.

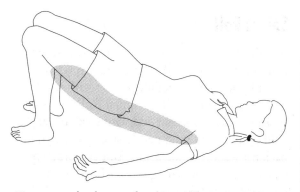

**Lie on your back, your feet hip-width apart and parallel, your arms by sides, and your hips lifted.**

3. As you exhale, slowly lower your spine to the floor one vertebrae at a time until your whole spine is resting on the floor. Relax for a few moments, feeling the natural curve at your lower back.

4. Repeat steps 1 through 3 three more times.

## Reclining Fork

You may remember the Reclining Fork from Chapter 7 as a way to address carpal tunnel syndrome. Now you'll use it to strengthen your back and abdominal muscles without straining your back. This stretch has been modified for your back by resting your forearms rather than your hands on the floor. Also, you'll be raising your chest as you exhale, not as you inhale.

1. Lie on your belly, with your forehead touching the floor. Place your forearms and palms flat on the floor so your arms are in a 90-degree position. Your elbows should line up with your shoulders, and your hands should line up with your elbows. Press the tops of your feet and your pubic bone into the floor. Notice how your lower back feels.

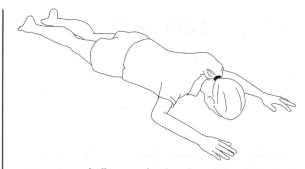

**Lie on your belly, your forehead touching the floor, your arms in a box position with your forearms and palms flat on the floor.**

2. As you exhale, slowly lift your chest off the floor, using your back muscles rather than your hands. Keep your mind on how your lower back feels as you lift your chest. Raise your chin slightly.

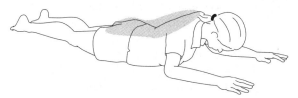

**Lie on your belly with your palms flat on the floor, your arms in a box position with your forearms and palms flat on the floor and your chest lifted.**

**Flex Alert!**

If you feel pain or tightness in your lower back as you lift your chest off the floor, raise your chest only to a point where you feel your back muscles contract. Stop at that point and then slowly lower your chest. Also use the strength of your arms to support your back by pressing your forearms lightly into the floor.

3. Hold the stretch as you inhale. Lower your chest to the floor as you exhale. Inhale with your chest on the floor. Lift your chest again as you exhale, hold your chest up as you inhale, and lower your chest as you exhale. Repeat these movements two more times. Hold the stretch

with your chest lifted off the floor for three breaths. Remember not to place any weight in your hands unless you feel tightness or strain in your back.

4. Release the stretch as you exhale. Rest and notice the results.

## Dragon's Tail

Dragon's Tail prevents and treats back soreness and sciatica by strengthening your abdominal muscles and back. As an added benefit, it helps release accumulated stress and enables you to unwind.

1. Lie on your belly, with your forehead touching the floor. Place your palms flat on the floor, under your shoulders. Roll your shoulders up toward your ears and down the back of your body, with your shoulder blades together and your elbows hugging your body. With your feet hip-width apart, press the tops of your feet and your pubic bone into the floor.

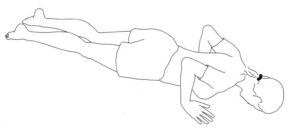

Lie on your belly with your forehead touching the floor, your palms flat on the floor under your shoulders, your elbows hugging your body, and the tops of your feet on the mat.

2. As you exhale, lengthen your right leg as if you're trying to touch the wall behind you and then slowly lift your leg off the floor. Feel your back muscles working while keeping your pelvis level. Do not roll your body to the side.

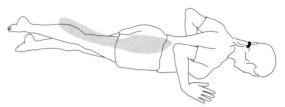

Lie on your belly with your forehead touching the floor, your palms flat on the floor under your shoulders, your elbows hugging your body, and your right leg lifted.

**S-t-r-e-t-c-h It Out**

Dragon's Tail is all about length, not height. Focus on keeping your leg lengthened rather than lifting it as high as possible. Keep your hipbones on the floor.

3. Inhale with your leg lifted, and slowly lower your leg as you exhale. Inhale while your legs are on the floor, and lengthen and lift your left leg as you exhale.

4. Repeat steps 2 and 3, alternating between your right and left legs, three more times. Rest and notice the results. If you feel any tension in your lower back, move to your hands and knees and practice the Z Stretch.

## The Least You Need to Know

◆ Four essential elements to include in your back-care program are relaxing your back, strengthening your abdominal muscles, stretching your hamstrings, and strengthening your back muscles.

◆ Stretching is one of the best relaxation techniques to nurse your back.

◆ Specific stretches, practiced regularly and safely, can cure sciatica.

◆ After you practice back strengthening stretches, be sure to relax and gently stretch your back.

# In This Chapter

- ◆ Uncover key times to work in stretching
- ◆ Reap the benefits of sports-related stretching
- ◆ The basics of stretching before or after sports
- ◆ Stretches to enhance sports participation and keep you strong and supple

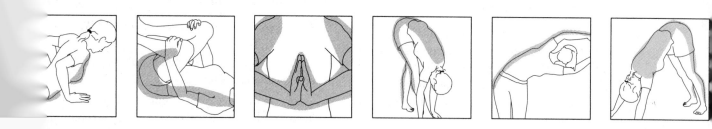

# Chapter 9

# Sports Stretching

Your exercise program should comprise three key elements: stretching, aerobic exercise, and strength training. Stretching not only prepares your body to work out by keeping your muscles limber, it also boosts your general conditioning and helps you maintain a full range of motion in your joints.

Every sport places particular demands on your body, and sport-specific stretching helps your muscles meet these demands. For example, if you play tennis or golf, practicing shoulder stretches loosens the muscles around your shoulder joint, making them supple and ready for action. Stretching may also decrease pain and soreness after exercise and reduce your risk of injury.

But which stretches should you master for sports, and when and how should you practice them? You'll find answers to these questions in this chapter. You learn how to stretch to keep yourself in "sports shape" with stretches designed to balance the effects of participating in certain sports. Discover, too, how to maintain balance if you play sports that may create imbalances between one side of your body and the other. You'll also follow recommendations about which types of sports to engage in, depending on your general health, and ways you can reduce your risk of sports-related injuries.

Armed with this knowledge, you'll be empowered to make wise decisions about when to practice specific stretches to receive the greatest benefits and when to avoid certain stretches that may exacerbate injuries. More important, you'll refine your sense of balance and coordination to reach new levels of performance excellence.

# Sports Stretching Basics

If you frequently participate in activities such as walking, running, hiking, cycling, swimming, tennis, or golf, you know how important it is to develop and maintain muscular strength and flexibility to keep you going strong. Stretching before and after vigorous activity is the best insurance to remain injury-free. It's easy, feels great, and doesn't cost a penny.

Sports that emphasize one side of your body, like golf, tennis, and baseball, may create imbalances between one side of your body and the other. For example, as you swing a golf club in one direction, you twist to one side of your body. Consequently, one side becomes strong but tight, while the other side becomes flexible but weak. Muscle imbalances may also result from repetitive motions. For instance, because running tends to use your hamstrings more than your quadriceps, your hamstrings become more powerful than your quadriceps, creating a common muscular imbalance.

When you stretch before, during, and after exercising, you may prevent injuries such as muscle strains and soreness. Warm up slowly and carefully before increasing the intensity of your workout. Ideally, you should stretch after you've warmed up at least 5 minutes and then hold each stretch for at least 30 seconds. The best time to stretch is after exercise, when your muscles are warm and more receptive to stretching; however, if you have time to stretch only once during your workout, stretch after you cool down.

**S-t-r-e-t-c-h It Out**

Stretching helps you cool down your body after vigorous exercise, to reduce any negative effects.

# Walking, Running, and Hiking

The symmetrical motions that occur when walking, running, and hiking provide many fundamental health benefits. These aerobic activities improve cardiovascular fitness, control weight, reduce blood pressure, increase circulation and respiration, and lower your resting heart rate.

A 30-minute daily walk is a great way to stay healthy. Running requires strength and endurance. And hiking, while resembling walking when on a flat terrain, can be more physically demanding when climbing and descending a hillside.

Before you begin any of these activities, practice a series of stretches that helps alleviate muscle stiffness and risk of pulled muscles. Upon your return, a cool-down stretch improves circulation and decreases buildup of *lactic acid.*

**Flexicon**

**Lactic acid** is a chemical byproduct that causes muscles to ache when exercised.

# Pyramid

Pyramid is an easy stretch to practice after you're warmed up. It's perfect for walkers, runners, and hikers because it stretches the hamstrings, which tend to get tight with repetitive movement. You'll also find Pyramid in Chapter 4.

1. Stand steadily on a firm surface, your feet even with your hips and your arms at your sides. Practice balance and coordination. Spreading your toes helps you establish a firm base of support. Gaze forward at one object to enhance your sense of balance.

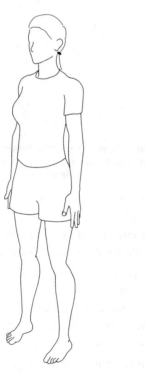

**Stand with your feet hip-width apart and your arms at your sides.**

2. Inhale as you step forward with your right foot, placing your right foot about a leg length in front of your left foot. Keep both legs straight with supple knees, feet flat on the floor, hips facing forward, weight even in both legs, arms by your sides.

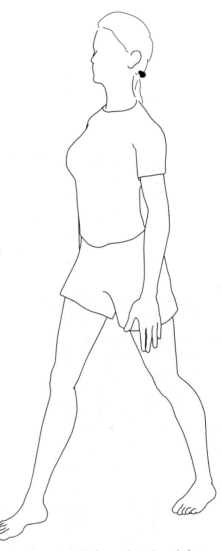

**Stand with your right foot a leg's length forward, your feet hip-width apart, and your arms by your sides.**

3. Raise both arms out to your sides and up by your ears as you inhale, palms turned toward one another. Drop your shoulders away from your ears. Keep your joints and muscles relaxed, and use envelope breathing. Pause.

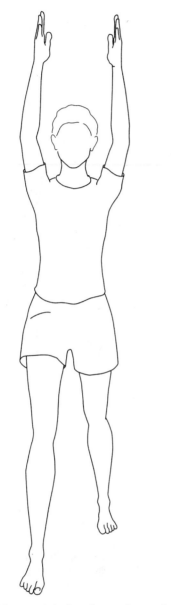

Stand with your right foot forward, your left leg back, and both arms up by your ears.

4. Sweep your arms out to the sides as you bend your torso forward toward your right thigh, placing your palms or fingers on either side of your right foot. Try to keep your right leg as straight as you comfortably can, bending your knee only as needed. Your back leg should remain straight.

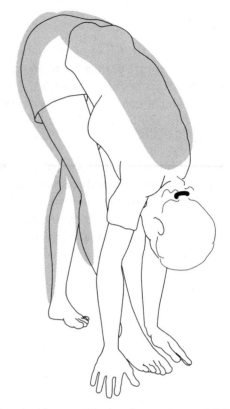

Stand with your right foot forward, your left leg back, and your palms on either side of your front foot.

5. Sweep your arms out to the sides as you inhale up to your standing position, and exhale as you bend forward again, placing your hands by your front foot.

6. Repeat steps 3 and 4 two more times, ending in the forward bending position. Hold the stretch for four deep breaths. The hip of your back leg should press outward away from your spine.

7. To release the stretch, glide your arms out to the sides as you inhale your torso up, and bring both arms to your sides as you exhale. Pause to rest for a moment.

8. Perform the Pyramid on the other side of your body by placing your left leg forward and right leg back, proceeding through steps 1 through 7. Observe any differences on this side of your body.

## One Leg Up, One Leg Down

You may remember One Leg Up, One Leg Down from Chapter 8. Practice this stretch after you exercise to receive the greatest benefits. It's also a great way to relax and unwind after your workout.

1. Lie on your back next to a doorframe or post. Exhaling, lift your left leg and place it against the doorframe or post, lengthening your right leg along the floor as you place your legs in a 90-degree position. Attempt to place your entire leg against the supporting surface. Bring your arms out from your body about 1 foot, with your palms turned up. Hold the stretch four deep breaths while maintaining a relaxed body.

2. Repeat the stretch with your right leg elevated.

**S-t-r-e-t-c-h It Out**

If you can't rest your whole leg on the supporting surface, keep practicing and enjoy moving closer to the 90-degree position.

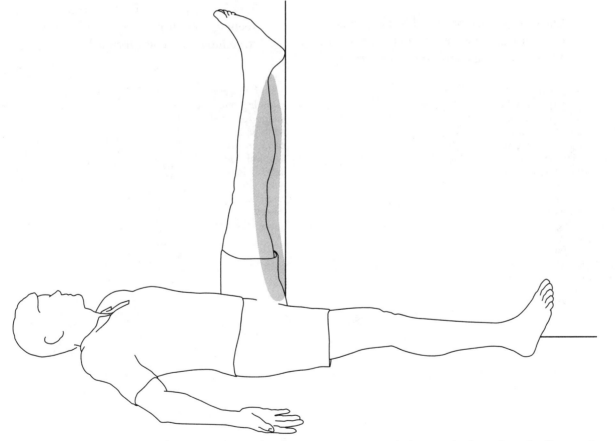

Lie on your back with your left leg placed on a doorframe or post, your right leg stretched out along the floor, and your arms out from your body with your palms turned up.

## Kneeling Hip Flexor Stretch

Remember your psoas muscle, defined in Chapter 4? The Kneeling Hip Flexor Stretch stretches your psoas and upper-thigh muscles that can get chronically tight if you regularly walk, run, or hike.

**Flex Alert!** _____

If you suffer from knee pain, proceed with caution when you try the Kneeling Hip Flexor Stretch. Skip this stretch if you experience sharp, shooting, or stabbing pain.

1. On a soft surface or folded blanket, kneel on your right knee. Keep your leg bent at a 90-degree angle and your knee directly below your right hip. Keep your left foot on the floor in front of you and your left knee bent directly over your left ankle at a 90-degree angle. Place your hands on your left thigh, and gaze forward.

2. Lunge forward, inhaling deeply into your chest, and stretch the front of your right thigh. Pause. As you exhale, return to the starting position (step 1).

3. Repeat steps 1 and 2 three more times. To stretch more deeply, bend your right knee and reach back with your right hand to hold your right ankle. Reach the left hand back as well if you can comfortably and steadily hold the stretch with one hand. Stay in this position for four deep breaths, keeping your arms straight and gently stretching your chest forward.

Stand with your right leg in a right angle, your knee below your right hip, your left foot on the floor in front of you, your left knee bent directly over your left ankle at a 90-degree angle, your hands on your left thigh, and gaze forward.

Stand on your right leg and lunge forward with your left knee in front of your left ankle, your chest expanded, and your gaze forward.

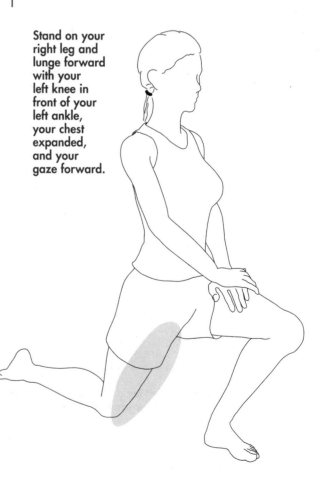

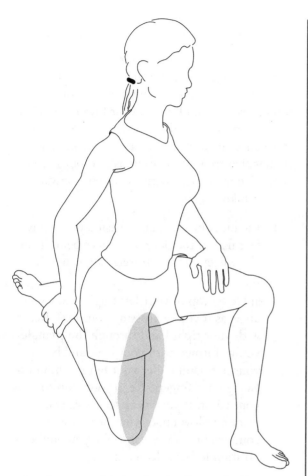

Stand on your right leg, lunging forward with your left knee in front of your left ankle, your chest expanded, and your hands holding your right ankle.

4. Repeat steps 1 through 3 on the other side of your body.

## Standing Quadriceps Stretch

This routine (also found in Chapter 4) is a great way to stretch quadriceps muscles overpowered by strong hamstrings. You may notice your walking and running stride lengthening when you make this stretch part of your before-and-after workout regimen. Keep your shoulders even and engage your abdominal muscles as you practice this stretch. And notice that you'll be applying the PNF stretching technique you learned in Chapter 2.

1. Stand tall, feet even with your hips, toes pointing forward. If it helps, steady yourself by holding on to a chair or placing your hand on a nearby wall.

2. Bend your right leg, and clasp your right foot with your right hand. Check your balance. Bring both knees toward one another, feeling the stretch in your right quadriceps.

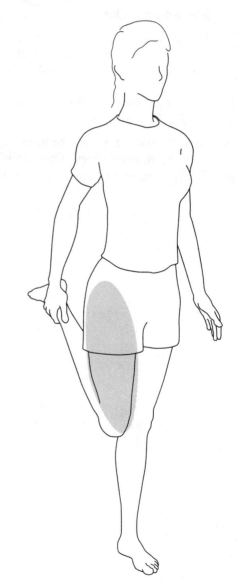

Stand with your feet hip-width apart, your right knee bent and your right hand holding your right foot.

3. Draw your ankle toward your buttocks. Now create resistance by applying the PNF stretch: simultaneously press the top of your foot into your hand and press your hand into your foot. Hold for one long, deep breath; relax the press; and hold the stretch for four breaths without the PNF press.

**S-t-r-e-t-c-h It Out** _____

Don't allow your knee to flare outward to the side. Keep your knees together.

4. Place your right foot back on the floor, and rest for three breaths.

5. Now stretch your right leg, repeating steps 1 through 4 two more times. Then stretch your left leg, repeating steps 1 through 4.

# Triangle Stretch with Moving Leg

Triangle Stretch with Moving Leg is similar to the Triangle Stretch in the "Hip and Knee Remedies" section of Chapter 7. The only difference is that you'll move your lower leg. This asymmetric stretch allows you to address muscle imbalances in your lower back, hips, and hamstrings that frequently occur as a response to repetitive movement patterns when you walk, run, or hike.

1. Lie on your back, arms beside your body, feet flat on the floor and knees bent. Take a few deep breaths to relax your muscles.

2. Pick up your right foot, placing your right ankle on top of your left thigh below your knee, as if you're crossing your legs. Reach with your right hand through the triangle you've formed with your legs, and bring your left hand under your left thigh, interlacing your fingers. Keep your chin toward your chest. If your neck feels strained, place a pillow under your head. Be as comfortable as you can while you hold this position for one deep breath.

Lie on your back with your right ankle on top of your left thigh below your knee, your hands clasped under your left thigh, your fingers interlaced, and your chin toward your chest.

**Flex Alert!** _____

If you suffer from knee pain or inflammation or you have recently had knee surgery, proceed with caution with this stretch. Stop if you experience pain as you move into the Triangle Stretch.

3. Lift your left foot toward the ceiling, straightening your left leg as you inhale. Pause to stretch your left hamstring. Bend your left knee as you exhale. Repeat these two movements three more times and then hold the stretch for four deep breaths with your knee bent and your lower leg relaxed.

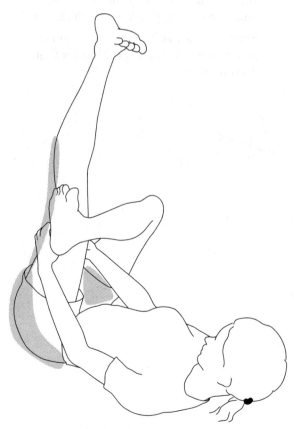

Lie on your back with your right ankle on top of your left thigh below your knee, your hands clasped under your left thigh, your fingers interlaced, your chin toward your chest, and your left leg straight with your foot lifted toward the sky.

4. Unwrap your legs and return to your starting position outlined in step 1. Take a few breaths and notice how your hips, back, and hamstrings feel and whether you experience any difference between the two sides.

5. Pick up your left foot, placing your left ankle on top of your right thigh below your knee, as if you're crossing your legs. Reach with your left hand through the triangle you've formed with your legs, and bring your right hand under your right thigh, interlacing your fingers. Keep your chin toward your chest. Hold the stretch one breath. Repeat step 3, this time stretching the right hamstring.

6. Return to your starting position, taking a few relaxing breaths.

**S-t-r-e-t-c-h It Out** _____

If you can't clasp your hands under your thigh, grab a strap. Place it under your thigh and hold either end of the strap with your hands. If you need to use a strap, do not practice the leg movement. Simply hold the stretch, as in the Triangle Stretch in Chapter 7.

# Cycling

Recreational and competitive cycling are popular and passionate sports. Cycling's benefits mirror those of running, walking, and hiking, and health-care professionals often recommend this low-impact sport as an alternative to the jarring motions of running.

Nevertheless, the constant movement of your hip joint can cause tight hip muscles, which may lead to problems such as a slower cadence. Muscle imbalances and tight muscles along the hips may result in lower-back pain. And shoulder, neck, and back tension may result from many hours spent hunched over handlebars.

# Z Stretch

Relax your back, shoulders, and hips after a long ride with the Z Stretch. This gentle stretch safely opens your hips. You may also notice its calming effects once you're finished with your ride.

**S-t-r-e-t-c-h It Out**

Use a firm folded blanket under your knees to protect these precious parts of your body.

1. Kneel on a blanket or rug with your knees placed directly beneath your hips and your shoulders positioned directly above your wrists. Spread your fingers wide, relax your shoulders, and inhale deeply into your chest, lifting your chin slightly at the top of the breath.

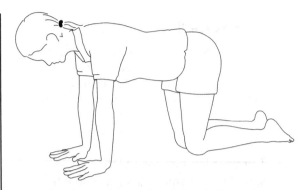

**Kneel with your knees placed directly beneath your hips, your shoulders positioned directly above your wrists, and your fingers spread.**

2. As you exhale, bring your chin toward your chest, your chest toward your thighs, and your hips toward your heels, moving into a crouching position like the letter Z.

3. Repeat steps 1 and 2 seven more times, and then rest in the Z position for four deep breaths.

**Kneel with your chin toward your chest, your chest toward your thighs, and your hips toward your heels.**

## Asymmetrical Hip Stretch

This stretch releases muscles surrounding your hip joints that are usually tight from cycling's repetitive motion. As an added benefit, you give your back and shoulders a well-deserved rest from supporting you on your bicycle. Have your mat ready to cushion your bones and a blanket handy to support your hip.

**Flex Alert!** _____

If you've recently had knee surgery or suffer from knee pain or inflammation, proceed with caution with this stretch.

1. Move to your hands and knees on your mat or a soft surface. Slide your right knee forward between your hands. Place your left hand on your right ankle and, without forcing it, move your lower right leg into a horizontal position (or as close to one as you can get). Place your hands under your shoulders and then slide your left leg back so it's straight.

2. Inhale deeply into your chest and hold your position. If there's space between your right hip and the floor, place your folded blanket underneath your hip to support it. If your body invites you to move into a deeper stretch, slowly lower your torso over your bent right leg, exhaling as you go, to a position you can sustain for a few breaths. Relax your upper body over your lower body. Concentrate on releasing any tension in the hip area as you remain in this position for four long, deep breaths.

3. To release the stretch, use your arms to lift your torso. Inhale deeply into your chest, expanding it toward your arms as you come up.

4. Move back to the starting position as in step 1. Bring your chest down to your thighs in a crouching position and rest for a few breaths. Notice how your hips feel.

5. Repeat steps 1 through 4, moving your left knee forward this time.

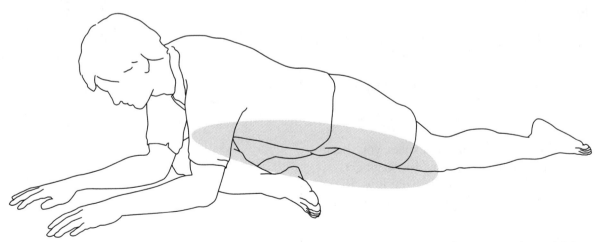

**Place your right knee forward between your hands, your lower right leg in a horizontal position, and your left leg lengthened back.**

# Swimming

Mainly an aerobic exercise, swimming is an outstanding rehabilitative activity. Because your body is supported by water, less stress is placed on your bones and joints. A great way to relax while you get a good full-body workout, swimming regularly builds endurance, muscle strength, and cardiovascular fitness.

Because your body is engaged in rhythmic motions, at times, swimming may cause some lower-back pain. The next four stretches help relax tight hip muscles that can hinder your ability to move through the water with ease.

## A Frame Stretch

The A Frame Stretch is versatile. You may remember it as a way to relieve headaches from Chapter 6. When you practice this stretch with your knees bent, you stretch your lower back and hips, which may be chronically tight from your swimming program.

**Flex Alert!** _____

Don't practice this stretch if you have uncontrolled high blood pressure; infection or inflammation of the eyes or ears; or chronic injury or inflammation of your back, legs, ankles, knees, hips, wrists, arms, or shoulders.

1. Move to your hands and knees, your hands below your shoulders with your fingers spread, your knees under your hips. Keep your shins and the tops of your feet on the floor. Kneel on a folded blanket to protect your knees, if you want to.

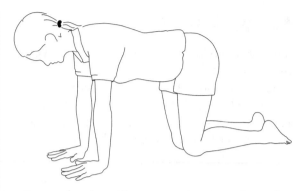

On your hands and knees, your hands are beneath your shoulders with your fingers spread, your knees under your hips, your shins and the tops of your feet on the floor.

2. Curl your toes, spread your fingers wide apart, and inhale deeply into your chest. Exhale as you press into your hands and feet to lift your hips. Keep your neck muscles relaxed and your knees bent. Keep breathing deeply. Hold this stretch for a few breaths, to allow your body to adjust to this position.

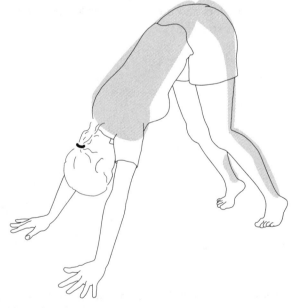

Your hands are on the floor with your fingers spread wide, your toes curled under, your hips up, and your knees bent.

3. Inhale, bend your right knee and exhale, press your left heel toward the floor. Inhale as you bend your left knee and then exhale and press your right heel toward the floor. Alternate these movements six to eight times.

4. Bring your knees to the floor as in step 1, and take a break.

5. Repeat step 2, moving back into the stretch, holding it, and breathing deeply for four breaths, if possible. Don't force or strain. Gradually work toward holding the A Frame Stretch for six to eight breaths. Remember to keep your head and neck relaxed.

**Your hands are on the floor with your fingers spread wide, your toes curled under, your hips up, and your left knee bent.**

**Your hands are on the floor with your fingers spread wide, your feet on the floor, and your hips up.**

# Diamond

Also found in Chapter 4, Diamond is a perfect stretch to loosen the muscles around your hip joint and inner thighs, two areas that tend to be chronically tight in swimmers.

1. Sit on a comfortable surface with a straight spine. Bring the soles of your feet together, your heels close to your groin, your legs in the shape of a diamond.

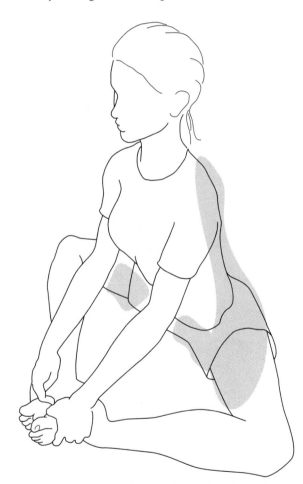

Sit with your knees bent and the soles of your feet together.

**S-t-r-e-t-c-h It Out** _____

Sit on the forward edge of a folded blanket to help keep your spine straight if your back is stiff or sensitive. If you have knee pain, kneel on folded blankets.

2. Hold your feet with your hands. If you feel your back rounding, hold your ankles or calves. Inhale deeply, and feel your spine elongate up toward the crown of your head. Keep your spine straight, your upper back flat, and your chin parallel to the floor. Move your feet away from your hips if you feel strain in your knees or groin. Don't force or strain!

3. Contract your abdominal muscles as you strongly exhale all your breath. It's okay if your body leans forward from the hips, but be sure you keep your back straight.

4. Hold this position for four long, smooth breaths, or even longer, if you want. Relax and let gravity do the work. Notice where you feel the stretch in your body.

## Ankles Alive

Bending your ankles keeps feet, ankles, and calves limber to enhance your swim. Perhaps you remember this stretch from Chapter 4. You can practice this effortless stretch anytime you can sit on the floor and lengthen your legs, perhaps immediately following your swim. Your ankle joints will thank you.

1. Sit on a folded blanket, if you need to, with your legs outstretched, your feet slightly apart, and your hands somewhat behind your buttocks. Use your arms to support your back as you lean backward a little.

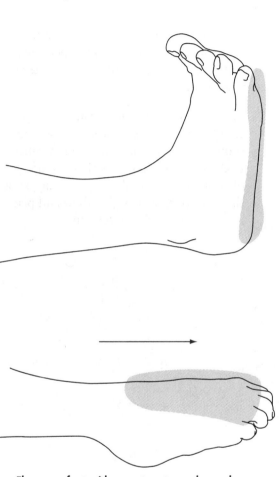

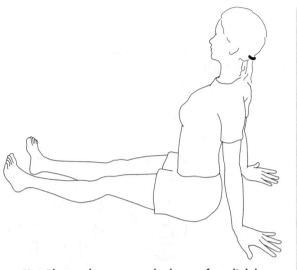

Sit with your legs outstretched, your feet slightly apart, your hands somewhat behind your buttocks, and lean back.

2. With your feet flexed and your toes pointed upward toward the sky, focus your attention on your ankles and feet. Inhaling, slowly flex your feet backward, bending them from the ankle joint and drawing them back toward your knees. Pause to hold this position. Exhale and then slowly move your feet forward, pointing your toes in an effort to touch the floor. Hold this position for a few seconds.

Flex your foot with your toes toward your knees and then point your foot with your toes away from your knees.

3. Repeat step 2 nine more times. Focus your attention on the stretch sensations, your breathing, and your count.

## Pretzel

Appearing also in Chapters 3 and 7, Pretzel is a perfect stretch for those tight upper-back and shoulder muscles that speak to you after a strenuous swim.

1. Sit in a sturdy chair on a firm seat with a straight spine. Keep your jaw loose, your shoulders relaxed, and your chin parallel to the floor. Straighten both arms in front of your torso at shoulder level, your palms skyward. Bend your right elbow and place it in the crease of your left elbow.

2. Entwine your arms until you can place the fingers of your left hand on your right palm. If you can't touch your fingers to your palm, bring them to your wrist or forearm in a loose wrap.

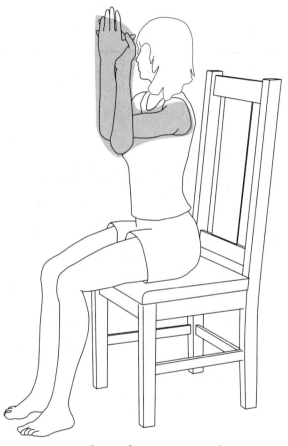

**Sit with your forearms entwined.**

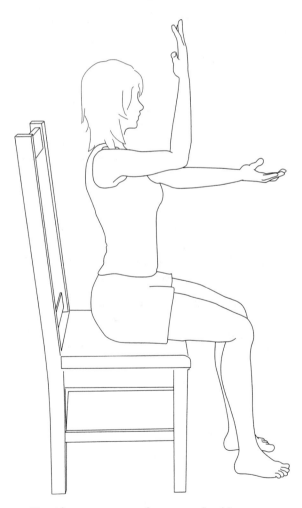

**Sit with your arms out from your shoulders, your right elbow at the crease of your left elbow.**

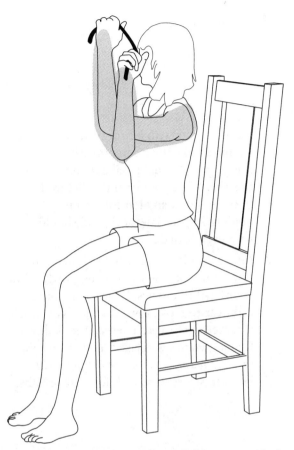

**Sit with your forearms entwined, holding one end of a strap in your left hand and grasping the other end with your right hand.**

3. Move your elbows up or down slowly until you find your edge, and hold the stretch for four deep breaths, sitting steady. Each time you inhale, imagine your upper back expanding. Picture your upper-back muscles becoming soft and pliable as you exhale. You may close your eyes to notice where you feel the stretch in your body.

4. Release your arms, let your hands rest on your thighs, and observe the difference in how your shoulders feel.

5. Repeat the steps, placing your left elbow in the crease of your right elbow, and once again hold your position for four breaths, noticing any variations as you stretch this side.

# Golf and Tennis

Golf and tennis are sports that emphasize one side of the body. Stretching both sides of your body evenly helps prevent problems that may occur because of imbalances created between one side of your body and the other.

In addition, the impact and stress of repetitive swinging motions can strain the muscles and joints in your lower back, elbows, shoulders, hands, and wrists. You may prevent injuries and increase your range of motion by stretching before and after you play. The next several stretches cover all the important body parts that need to be stretched to keep you flexible and strong for your game.

## Wrist Waves

Perhaps you remember Wrist Waves from the "Wrists and Hands" section in Chapter 3. A great stretch for your forearm muscles and wrist joints, it wards off muscle soreness and joint pain that may occur after a long day of golf or tennis.

1. Sit in a heavy chair and keep your spine straight. Firmly plant your feet directly under your knees. Raise your arms in front of your torso at shoulder level, with your palms down toward the floor. Bend your hands backward, your fingers pointing upward, as if you were gesturing "stop." Inhale and then pause to feel the stretch.

2. Bend your hands forward, your fingers pointing downward as you exhale.

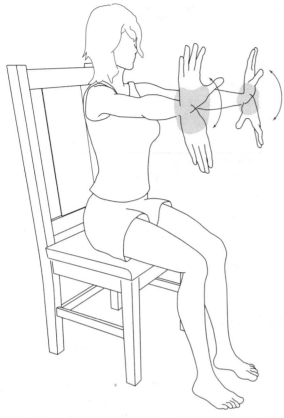

Sit with your arms stretched forward at shoulder level, your palms up and then down.

3. Repeat steps 1 and 2 nine more times, breathing and counting as you move. Keep your fingers and elbows straight, your fingers together, and your palms open as if you are waving. If your arms tire, take a break and rest your hands on your thighs. Focus your mind on the movement of your wrist joint, stretch sensations, your breathing, and counting.

## Seated Neck Stretch

After a long stretch of golf or a challenging tennis match, take a seat, relax, and give the small muscles of your neck a rest as you stretch and lengthen them. The Seated Neck Stretch is also found in Chapter 6.

**Flex Alert!** _____

If you suffer from neck injury or pain, stretch with care, especially if your pain increases or you feel numbness.

1. Sit on a chair with a firm seat, your spine straight. Take three long breaths, feeling the length of your spinal column as you breathe. With your chin parallel to the floor, let go of any tension you may be holding in your jaw, neck, and shoulders with every exhale.

2. Inhale deeply and gently lift your head toward the sky. As you exhale, slowly allow your head to move sideways and your right ear to move toward your right shoulder. Keep your eyes open and look down, keeping your jaw relaxed. *Do not raise your shoulder toward your ear or lift your chin.* Hold this passive stretch for four breaths.

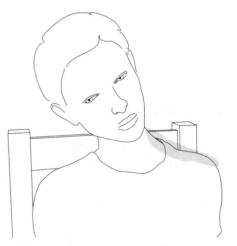

Sit on a chair with your spine straight, your right ear toward your right shoulder, and your eyes open and looking down.

3. Repeat step 2, this time allowing your left ear to move toward your left shoulder. Practice two more sets.

# Ankle Circles

Ankle Circles, which made its debut in Chapter 4, helps protect your vulnerable ankles from the effects of high-impact sports such as tennis and the bending and twisting motions in golf. You'll lubricate your ankle joint; stretch your calves, ligaments, and tendons; and strengthen weak muscles in this area.

1. Sit with your legs outstretched, your feet slightly apart, your hands somewhat behind your buttocks, on a folded blanket if you need to. Use your arms to support your back as you lean back a little. Alternatively, you could lie on your back with your legs raised.

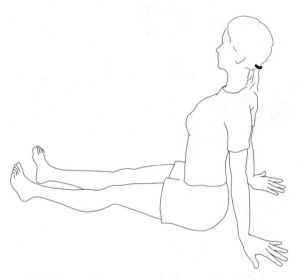

**Sit with your legs outstretched, your feet slightly apart, your hands somewhat behind your buttocks, and lean back.**

2. Keep your legs separated but straight and your heels on the ground if you're sitting. Rotate your left foot clockwise 10 times and then counterclockwise 10 times. Inhale as you move your foot up, and exhale as you move it down. Pay close attention to the circling motion, closing your eyes to avoid distraction. Notice the range of motion in each ankle as you move.

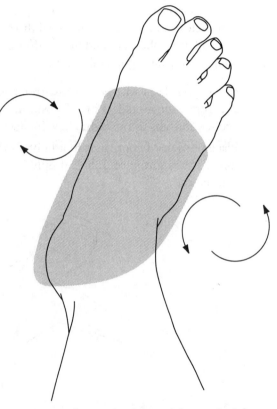

**Rotate your foot to the right and then to the left.**

3. Repeat step 2 with your right foot. Bring both feet together and rotate them at the same time clockwise 10 times and then counterclockwise 10 times.

4. Finally, separate your feet and rotate them 10 times in one direction and then 10 times in the opposite direction.

# Reclining Twist

Practice the Reclining Twist so you can swing your racket or golf club with ease. Rotating, extending, and aligning your spinal column increases the circulation of blood and oxygen to your muscles and hydrates your spinal discs. You'll also alleviate shoulder and neck stiffness that often accompanies golf and tennis.

1. Lie on your back with your arms stretched out from your shoulders in a *T* position. Scoot your hips to the right a few inches.

2. Place the sole of your right foot lightly on top of your right knee. Inhale deeply into your chest.

3. Twist your torso to the left, and as you exhale, bring your right knee toward your left hand and turn your head to the right.

4. Unwind your torso back to the starting position as you inhale.

5. Repeat steps 3 and 4 three more times. Then hold the twist for four deep breaths.

6. Repeat the twist on the other side of your body.

 **Flex Alert!** _____

Do not practice the Reclining Twist if your back is sore or injured.

Lie on your back with your arms stretched out from your shoulders in a T position, the sole of your right foot on top of your right knee, your torso twisted to the left, your right knee toward your left hand, and your head turned to the right.

# Standing Squat

Golf and tennis place huge demands on your back, hips, and legs. Hips tighten, causing loss of mobility, which can affect your gait and swing. Constant walking, running, and lunging place pressure on your lower back and knee joints. The Standing Squat addresses all these issues and strengthens the muscles that surround your knee joints.

**Flex Alert!** _____

Don't practice the Standing Squat if you're suffering from knee pain or injury. Never force or strain.

1. Stand, with your feet even with your hips, your toes pointing forward, and your arms at your sides.

2. Lift your arms forward and up at shoulder level, with your palms down, as you inhale.

3. Slowly squat, and as you exhale, bend your knees forward over your ankles until your thighs are parallel with the floor. If your thighs cannot move to this parallel position, simply move them to a position that feels comfortable.

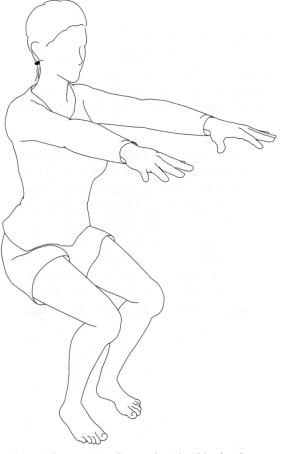

Squat with your arms forward at shoulder level, your palms down, your knees forward over your ankles, and with your thighs parallel to the floor.

4. Slowly straighten your legs as you inhale.

5. Repeat steps 3 and 4 three more times, and then hold the squat for three deep breaths.

6. Repeat step 4 to come out of the stretch.

## Puppy Stretch

The Puppy Stretch loosens tight muscles between the shoulder blades that may have become overtaxed from swinging your racket or club. It also opens up your armpits, neck, and chest. Practice Puppy in the evening to ensure restful sleep.

1. Kneel on a mat or blanket, placing your hands beneath your shoulders and your knees beneath your hips. Inhale deeply, and as you exhale, slide your palms forward to a point where you feel a nice stretch in your armpits and chest. Your arms should be straight, but if you need to, you may keep a slight bend in your elbows. Allow your head to rest on the mat or blanket, and let your neck relax.

2. Hold the stretch for four deep breaths. As you inhale, feel your chest expand. As you exhale, apply a little pressure to your *sternum*, pressing your chest toward the floor while your hips remain upward toward the sky.

> **Flexicon**
>
> Commonly called the breastbone, your **sternum** is a long, flat bone in the center of your chest. Connected to your ribs with cartilage, the sternum protects your lungs and heart.

3. Come out of the stretch by moving your hands back to the starting position, under your shoulders, as you come to your hands and knees. Sit back on your heels, if you can, and notice how your shoulders, neck, and chest feel.

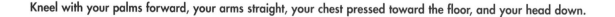

**Kneel with your palms forward, your arms straight, your chest pressed toward the floor, and your head down.**

# Standing Quadriceps Stretch

The popular and effective Standing Quadriceps Stretch appears in the "Walking, Running, and Hiking" section of this chapter and also in Chapter 4. By stretching the front of your body, this routine counteracts the stress on your knees caused by twisting and bending forward while playing golf and tennis. Don't forget to engage your abdominal muscles and keep your shoulders even as you practice this stretch. And don't forget to apply the PNF technique described in Chapter 2.

1. Stand tall, your feet even with your hips, your toes pointing forward. If it helps, steady yourself by holding on to a chair or placing your hand on a nearby wall.

2. Bend your right leg and clasp your right foot with your right hand. Check your balance. Bring both knees toward one another, feeling the stretch in your right quadriceps.

3. Draw your ankle toward your buttocks. Now create resistance by applying the PNF stretch: simultaneously press the top of your foot into your hand and press your hand into your foot. Hold for one long, deep breath; relax the press; and hold the stretch for four breaths without the PNF press.

**S-t-r-e-t-c-h It Out** _____
Don't allow your knee to flare outward to the side. Keep your knees together.

4. Place your right foot back on the floor, and rest for three breaths.

5. Now stretch your right leg, repeating steps 1 through 4 two more times. Then stretch your left leg, repeating steps 1 through 4.

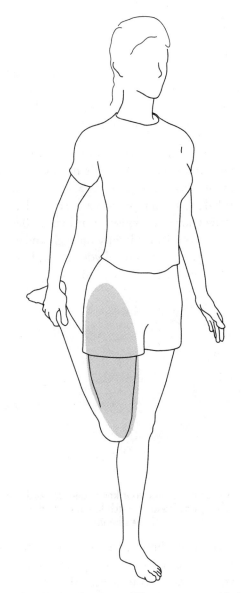

**Stand with your feet hip-width apart, your right knee bent, with your right hand holding your right foot.**

**A Stretch in Time ...** _____
Work the Standing Quadriceps Stretch into your day: on your way out the door to work in the morning and as you arrive in the evening, use the doorway to support you as you stretch.

# Knee Press

Golf and tennis place a huge demand on your back and hips. The Knee Press, which made its debut in Chapter 8, releases your tired back, gently soothes aching hips, and, as an added benefit, strengthens your abdominal muscles.

1. Lie on your back on a comfortable surface (not your bed). Inhale deeply. As you exhale, draw one knee toward your chest. Inhale again, and with the next exhale, draw your other knee toward your chest. Place your hands lightly on each knee. Tuck your chin toward your chest, but keep your head on the floor.

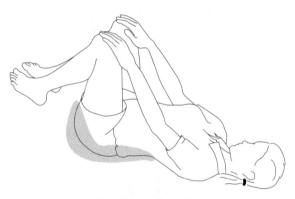

**Lie on your back with your knees bent toward your chest, one hand on each knee, and your elbows bent.**

2. Move your thighs away from your chest as you inhale and straighten your arms. Keep your hands on your knees. Move your thighs toward your chest, bending your elbows as you exhale. Do not pull or force your legs toward your chest. Practice these movements eight times.

**Flex Alert!** _____

Step 3 of the Knee Press is more strenuous than steps 1 and 2. Do not practice step 3 if you have had recent abdominal surgery or if you experience pain after trying one repetition.

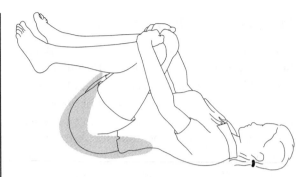

**Lie on your back with your knees bent toward your chest, one hand on each knee, and your arms straight.**

3. With your head resting on the floor, grasp your arms around your knees to form your body into a ball. Hold on to your hand, wrist, or forearm as you draw your knees toward your chest. Rest your head on the floor. Take one deep, full breath in this position. Inhale, and as you exhale, bring your nose toward your knees, engaging your abdominal muscles as you move.

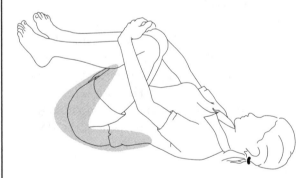

**Lie on your back with your knees bent, your arms wrapped around your legs, and your head on the floor.**

4. Lower your upper back to the floor and relax your shoulders as you inhale. Repeat these movements two more times, then rest with your hands on your knees for a few moments.

## Standing Chest Stretch

The Standing Chest Stretch reverses the effects of swinging your racket or club—in particular, rounding your upper and back and shoulders. Your abdominal muscles, chest, shoulders, arms, hands, and fingers are all stretched simultaneously.

**S-t-r-e-t-c-h It Out**

Have a rolled-up bath towel or strap handy for this stretch. If you can't interlace your fingers after sweeping your arms toward your back, clasp the strap or towel with both hands.

1. Stand on a firm surface with your feet a little wider than your hips. Bend your knees slightly. Let your arms rest by your sides.

2. As you inhale, lift your arms forward and up to the level of your shoulders. Stretch through your fingertips with your palms down.

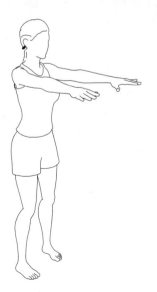

Stand on a firm surface with your feet a little wider than hip-width apart, your arms forward at shoulder level with your palms down, and stretch through your fingertips.

3. Circle your arms out to the sides and behind your back, turning your palms toward one another. Exhale as you interlace your fingers. Squeeze your palms together if you can, pressing your knuckles down and back. Or firmly hold the ends of your strap or towel. Your arms should be as straight as possible, with each shoulder blade moving toward the other and your sternum pressed forward to open your chest.

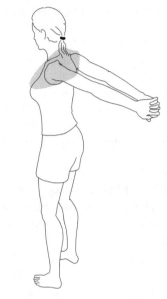

Stand with your arms straight behind your back at shoulder level, your palms together and your sternum pressed forward.

4. Hold the stretch for four deep, full breaths. As you inhale, you may lift your arms toward the sky to move deeper into the stretch. Relax the intensity of the stretch as you exhale.

5. Relax your arms beside your body, and rest to feel the effects of the stretch.

**A Stretch in Time ...**

Try practicing the Standing Chest Stretch while you're waiting in line or anytime you feel the need to pass the time with an activity.

# Lunging Forward and Back

Target your hips, hamstrings, calves, back, and neck with this dynamic stretch. Holding the stretch in different positions targets those hard-to-reach areas that may become imbalanced or tight from repetitively swinging your tennis racket or golf club. Opening your hips and stretching your legs and back helps you move more easily during your game. Lunging Forward and Back is similar to the Runner's Stretch found in the "Hip Openers" section of Chapter 4.

**S-t-r-e-t-c-h It Out**

Gather your mat or kneel on a rug, and have a blanket handy to protect your precious knees.

1. Move to your hands and knees on a soft surface or blanket. Step your right foot forward between your hands, with your knee over your ankle and your shin straight. Extend your left leg backward, knee down, with the top of your left foot on the floor. Place your hands directly beneath your shoulders to support your upper body.

2. Draw in a deep breath. As you exhale, slowly begin to straighten your right leg, moving your hips back over your left heel until you feel a nice stretch in your right hamstring. Move your hands back toward your hips, using your arms to support you as you move. Rest your torso forward toward your right thigh.

3. Slowly come back to the starting position as you inhale.

4. Repeat steps 2 and 3 two more times, and then hold the forward lunge for four deep breaths, allowing your hips to sink with every exhale. Gaze forward or look down to relax the back of your neck. Protect your vulnerable knees by keeping your right knee over your right ankle. Optimally, place your palms on either side of your front foot; if that doesn't work for you, make fists with your hands.

5. Repeat step 2, bringing your body to the hamstring stretch position. Hold this stretch for four deep breaths.

6. Repeat step 3 and then move back to your hands and knees. Repeat steps 1 through 5 with your left leg forward and right leg back.

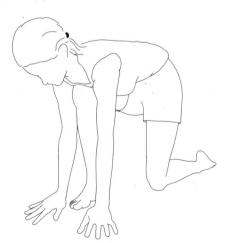

**Lunge with your right foot forward and your left leg back.**

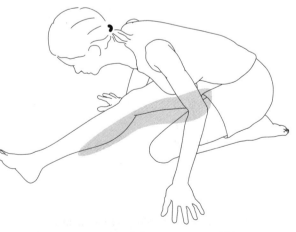

**Lunge with your right leg straight, your hips over your left heel, and your hands back toward your hips.**

## The Least You Need to Know

◆ Always stretch after you've warmed up at least 5 minutes to increase your range of motion.

◆ Stretch again after you've cooled down; however, if you have time to stretch only once during your workout, stretch *after* you exercise.

◆ Stretching can lessen the pain and soreness you may feel after a strong workout.

◆ Stretching helps remediate muscle imbalances that may occur from stressing a particular part of the body, such as the effects of twisting your body in one direction when playing baseball and golf.

# In This Chapter

- ◆ Stay healthy and vital with physical activity

- ◆ Senior-friendly types of physical activities

- ◆ A review of essential safety tips

- ◆ Easy-to-follow seated and standing stretch routines
  that add strength, flexibility, and balance to your life

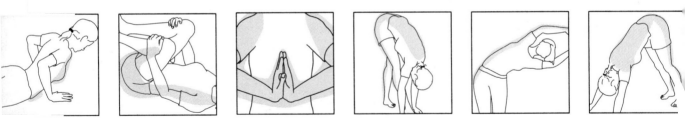

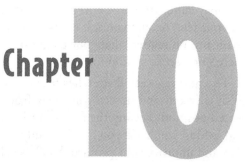

Chapter **10**

# Seniors' Stretch

You're wise enough to know how important it is to keep moving as you age. Your body was made to move, and activity helps your body run smoothly by keeping bones, muscles, and joints healthy and flexible. Maintaining the full range of motion through your joints keeps you in better balance. Stiffness results from inactivity and a sedentary lifestyle, not aging.

Maintaining endurance, strength, and flexibility is imperative for seniors who want to preserve strong muscles and bones. Including a regular stretching routine in your exercise program gives you more freedom of movement to do the things you need, want, and like to do. Remember, though, that although stretching exercises alone can improve your flexibility, they won't improve your endurance or strength.

If you're able, engage in cardiovascular exercises such as walking, swimming, or cycling, and strengthening exercises such as lifting light weights. Stretching is a great alternative, however, if strength and cardiovascular exercises are not an option for you.

Even if you have suffered from illness, surgery, or injury, in this chapter you'll find specific stretches to practice if you're recovering or have low energy. As you stretch, you'll develop body awareness and improve your posture. You'll employ tools to prevent rounded upper backs and nasty falls. And you'll learn how to sit correctly and stretch your body from a seated position, to breathe deeply for extra energy and enhanced relaxation, and to practice coordination and balance skills to prevent injury from falling.

It's time to be strong, flexible, and steady. So have some fun as you engage in these easy-to-follow seated and standing stretch routines that add strength, flexibility, and balance to your life.

# Sit and Stretch

If you're recovering from an illness or injury, you may suffer from low energy, feel unsteady on your feet, or find yourself confined to a chair. But no matter what your condition, there's no excuse to stop moving.

The next few seated stretches teach you how to sit correctly and stretch your body from a seated position. Feeling the firm chair beneath and behind you helps you develop body awareness and improve your posture. You'll receive many of the same benefits as in standing or reclining stretches, and best of all, when you're tired, you won't have to travel far to stop and rest.

### A Stretch in Time ...

Stretching cold muscles may cause injury, so always take the time to warm up before stretching. Stretch either before or after an easy walk. If you can't engage in endurance or strength exercises, stretch at least three times a week, moving slowly and relaxing as you go.

## Seated Chest Expander

The Seated Chest Expander is a simple stretch you can practice no matter how you feel. Sitting straight on a sturdy chair helps you lengthen your spinal column so you can breathe more deeply and expand your lungs. You'll become more aware of your posture, to prevent a rounded upper back. Extending your arms to the sides strengthens your chest, shoulders, and arms. Deep breathing relaxes you so you can rest more easily. When you're finished, you'll feel full of life, energy, and strength.

### Flex Alert!

Stretching should never cause pain. If you feel pain as you stretch, you've gone past your edge and need to back off. Remember that mild discomfort or a mild pulling sensation is normal.

1. Sit upright on a firm, stable seat with a backrest. Place your feet even with your hips. Position your hips, knees, and ankles at a 90-degree angle. If your feet don't reach the floor, put a cushion under your feet so they can rest firmly on the floor.

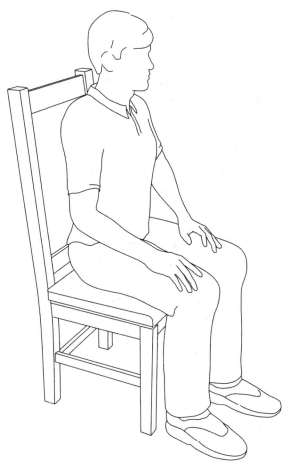

Sit upright on a firm seat with a backrest with your feet hip-width apart and your hips, knees, and ankles at a 90-degree angle.

2. Place one palm over the other at the center of your chest. Open your arms wide and inhale, expanding your lungs. Continue opening your arms as wide as you comfortably can without causing strain or discomfort. Exhale, and return your hands back to the starting position, palm over palm.

### S-t-r-e-t-c-h It Out

Focus your attention on breathing into the lower lobes of your lungs. Feel the back of your lungs expanding in your middle back. Don't forget to use envelope breathing.

3. Repeat step 2 five additional times. With each progressive repetition, feel your breath expanding with each inhale and deepening with your exhale. Notice the relaxing component of deep breathing.

### Flex Alert!

Avoid using your neck, jaw, or upper shoulder muscles—keep them relaxed. Be sure you're sitting in an upright posture throughout the stretch. Feel free to rest between repetitions to catch your breath or to relax your muscles if you need to.

**Now stretch your arms out to the side.**

# Seated Twist

The Seated Twist is a great stretch for posture. With it, you strengthen and realign your spinal column and add flexibility to your back. Twisting also massages your liver, stomach, spleen, pancreas, kidneys, and digestive tract. And with practice, you'll strengthen your abdominal muscles.

1. Sit upright on a firm, stable seat with a backrest. Place your feet even with your hips. Position your hips, knees, and ankles at a 90-degree angle. Be sure you're seated in the middle of the chair so you have room to move. Sit tall, with your palms facing down on your lap. If your feet don't reach the floor, put a cushion under your feet so they can rest firmly on the floor.

2. Inhale, and raise your arms up and out to your side so they're even with your shoulders. Twist your trunk to the right until your shoulders are parallel with your right thigh. Place your left hand on your right thigh, keeping your right hand comfortably behind the chair. Exhale. Do not force the twist. Instead, move gently as you turn from facing forward to the side. Inhale as you return to the center, and exhale as you move into the twist.

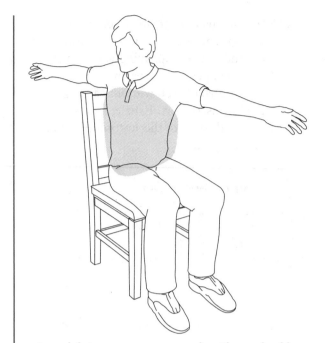

Seated, bring your arms out to the sides at shoulder height and twist your trunk to the right.

3. Repeat step 2 four times, alternating on each side. Work up to six repetitions, if you want, but be gentle with the twist. If you feel steady and your breath is relaxed, you may choose to stay in the twist four to six breaths.

### S-t-r-e-t-c-h It Out

Avoid the tendency to use your hands to force your body into the twist. Feel the twist begin as you exhale, and draw your navel toward your spine. Focus your attention on practicing slow, relaxing breaths.

### Flex Alert!

If you've had a hip replacement, don't bend your hips past a 90-degree angle. Never "bounce" into a stretch, but move slowly and steadily. Always keep a slight bend in your knees, shoulders, elbows, and hips as you stretch, and keep your joints relaxed.

## Seated Forward Bend

Here's a great stretch if your back feels tight and you've been sitting for a long time, whether at work or while traveling. If you have trouble sleeping, move into the forward bend before you retire, and relax in restful slumber.

1. Sit upright on a firm, stable seat with a backrest. Place your feet even with your hips. Position your hips, knees, and ankles at a 90-degree angle. Be sure you're seated in the middle of the chair so you have room to move. Sit tall, using your strong back muscles to maintain an upright posture. If this position is difficult for you, lean against the back of the chair. If your feet don't reach the floor, put a cushion under your feet so they can rest firmly on the floor.

2. Inhale deeply, feeling your lungs expand in all areas of your chest and middle back. As you exhale, slowly slide your hands down the front of your legs until you feel a gentle stretch in your back. Inhale as you return to the starting position, sitting as tall as you possibly can. Move forward on the exhale. Repeat these movements six times.

3. If you feel stable and your breath is even, hold the forward bend for six breaths.

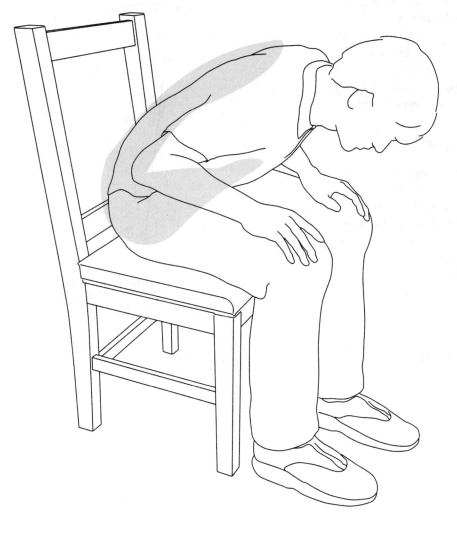

Sit in a chair with your upper body folded over your lower body.

# Standing Your Ground

You know that weight-bearing exercise is important for seniors to maintain strong muscles and bones. Steadiness and balance are key factors in preventing falls. Consequently, it's vital to engage daily in standing activities.

Make these standing balance exercises part of your morning routine. Each time you "stand your ground," you'll develop and refine your sense of balance. Checking your sense of balance is a wise general health check. As you tune into your body's natural ability to balance itself, you may notice day-to-day differences that provide clues to your general health. When you're rested and healthy, your balance is strong; when you're tired or ill, your balance is weak. This signal helps you make the right decisions, such as resting when you feel "under the weather." Once you become adept at standing your ground with your eyes open, you can challenge yourself by standing with your eyes closed.

## Standing Balance Exercise: Part 1

Great for balance and increasing confidence in seniors who have fallen or are at risk of falls, the two Standing Balance Exercises also strengthen your body. This first weight-bearing stretch fine-tunes your balance and strengthens the large muscles and bones that support your torso. It's time to add balance and strength to your life. Enjoy the feeling of being in balance and centered.

1. Stand tall, with your feet even with your hips and your toes pointing forward on a flat, even surface. Focus your eyes on a point in front of you. Keep your arms relaxed at your sides. The top of your head should feel as if it's stretching toward the sky. Your feet should feel like the strong roots of a tree.

2. Inhale and shift your weight forward onto the balls of your feet. Exhale and shift your weight backward onto your heels. Move comfortably with your breath in a safe range of motion. Keep your spine erect as you lean forward and back. Start with a small range of movement and then add more movement as your confidence and trunk stability increase.

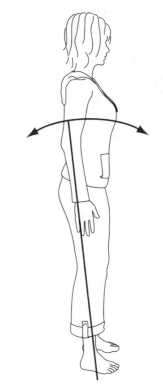

Stand with your feet hip-width apart and shift your weight forward toward the balls of your feet and then backward toward your heels.

**Flex Alert!**

For added stability, place your feet wider than your hips, and stand with your back close to a wall or support yourself by placing your hand on the wall. Avoid raising your heels as you lean forward or lifting your toes as you lean backward.

## Standing Balance Exercise: Part 2

Standing Balance Exercise: Part 2 has the same benefits as the first exercise with the same name. This time, though, you go side to side instead of forward to back.

1. Stand tall, with your feet even with your hips and your toes pointing forward on a flat, even surface. Focus your eyes on a point in front of you. Keep your arms relaxed at your sides. The top of your head should feel as if it's stretching toward the sky. Your feet should feel like the strong roots of a tree.

2. Inhale and shift your weight to your right leg. Exhale as you shift to the center. Pause and inhale as you feel a sense of stability. Exhale and shift your weight to your left leg.

3. Repeat these movements side to side, alternating sides, 12 times total. Remember to breathe with your movements, stand tall, and move in comfortable ranges of motion. Slowly start to increase your range of movement as your confidence and trunk stability increase.

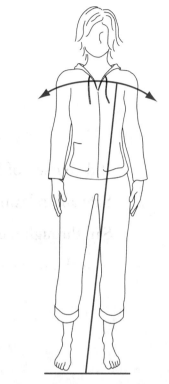

Stand with your feet hip-width apart and shift your body side to side.

### S-t-r-e-t-c-h It Out

If you like challenges, stand on thick carpet, a cushion, or a pillow. Need more support? Stand with your back against the wall. Keep your head always aligned upright, looking straight. Your risk of falling increases if your head is excessively forward or you look down. Your head weighs 10 pounds, so keep it upright and aligned with the rest of your body.

## The Least You Need to Know

◆ Stretching is a healthful and safe alternative to immobility.

◆ You can keep moving even if you are confined to a chair by enjoying safe seated stretches.

◆ Stretching helps improve your posture so you can breathe deeply and feel more alive and energetic.

◆ Warm up before you stretch, either after endurance and strength exercises or after an easy walk.

◆ If stretching is your primary means of exercise, be sure you stretch three times a week.

◆ Balancing exercises are your best and cheapest insurance against nasty falls.

# In This Chapter

- ◆ Rid yourself of PMS symptoms naturally
- ◆ Safe and relaxing stretches for the mother-to-be
- ◆ Sail through menopause by stretching
- ◆ Stretch away stress and find a new you

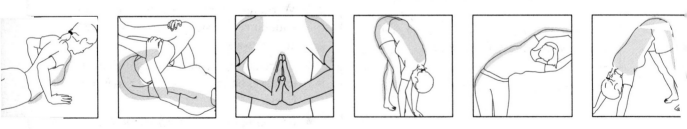

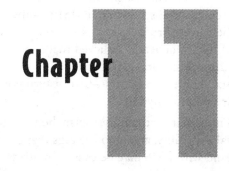

# Chapter 11

# Just for Her

Let's face it ladies, you know how much you give; now it's time to receive. If you nurture yourself at every stage of your life, you'll be happy you did. Listen to your body and give it what it needs during the key stages in your life as a woman.

Empower yourself with the tools you need to eliminate symptoms of PMS—the irritability, mood swings, frazzled nerves, mild backache, and anxiety. The way you live your life can greatly affect your chances of experiencing PMS. Don't wait until PMS strikes—start stretching now, and you'll be amazed by the results. Relax away symptoms of PMS and release stress by stretching your body.

Feel prepared as you stretch your way through pregnancy and the birth of your baby. Stretch safely throughout your pregnancy so you and your growing baby can enjoy each day and feel confident. In this chapter, you also learn stretches to practice at different stages of your pregnancy.

As you gracefully meet menopause, you can significantly influence your likelihood of becoming intimate with its symptoms. Take a moment to pause as you incorporate stretching into your daily routine. Use this pivotal time to reflect, relax, and release stress by stretching your body.

The simple act of stretching your body can release hidden stress and tension so you can live happily. You know stress is inherent in your life, so start managing your stress through stretching by learning about common body parts where stress is stored. And employ stretches to develop body awareness so you can respond to daily strains and ward off stress-related illnesses such as heart disease, cancer, and stroke.

# PMS

Most women experience one or more symptoms of premenstrual syndrome (PMS) at some point in their lives. Precisely why is still unknown, although it's generally believed that a major contributor is hormonal imbalance—often caused by lifestyle factors—that disturb your body's natural rhythms.

The anxiety, irritability, melancholy, emotional instability, and mood swings that go hand in hand with PMS may be caused by stress, poor eating habits, traveling, overwork, difficulties in relationships, and lack of exercise. These symptoms, as well as physical symptoms such as bloating, breast tenderness, food cravings, headaches, and weight gain, may be relieved by practicing specific stretches designed to provide immediate relief from the discomfort of PMS. Adding a diligent stretching program to your daily routine enables you to rid yourself of this nagging syndrome so you can relax and enjoy your life.

## A Frame Stretch

The A Frame Stretch is "flexible." Perhaps you've used it as a way to relieve headaches (Chapter 6) or loosen tight hips from swimming (Chapter 9). In this context, the A Frame Stretch helps you say good-bye to the irritability and anxiety that arrive with PMS.

 **Flex Alert!**

If you have uncontrolled high blood pressure; infection or inflammation of the eyes or ears; or chronic injury or inflammation of your back, legs, ankles, knees, hips, wrists, arms, or shoulders, don't practice this stretch.

1. Move to your hands and knees, with your hands below your shoulders, your fingers spread, and your knees under your hips. Keep your shins and the tops of your feet on the floor. Kneel on a folded blanket to protect your knees, if you need to.

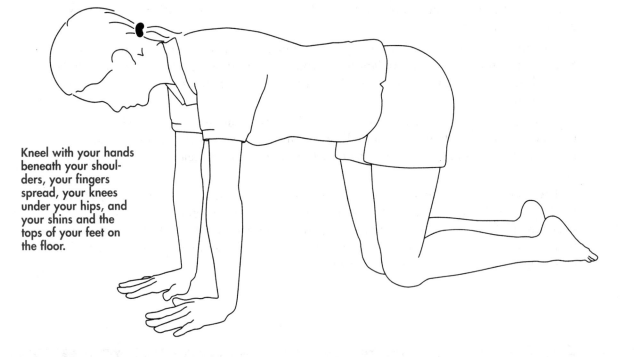

Kneel with your hands beneath your shoulders, your fingers spread, your knees under your hips, and your shins and the tops of your feet on the floor.

2. Curl your toes, spread your fingers wide apart, and inhale deeply into your chest. Exhale as you press into your hands and feet to lift your hips. Keep your neck muscles relaxed and your knees bent. Keep breathing deeply. Hold this stretch for a few breaths, to allow your body to adjust to this position.

3. Inhale, bend your right knee and exhale, press your left heel toward the floor. Inhale as you bend your left knee and exhale press your right heel toward the floor. Alternate these movements six to eight times.

4. Bring your knees to the floor as in step 1, and take a break.

5. Repeat step 2, moving back into the stretch, holding it and breathing deeply for four breaths, if possible. Don't force or strain. Gradually work toward holding the A Frame Stretch for six to eight breaths. Remember to keep your head and neck relaxed.

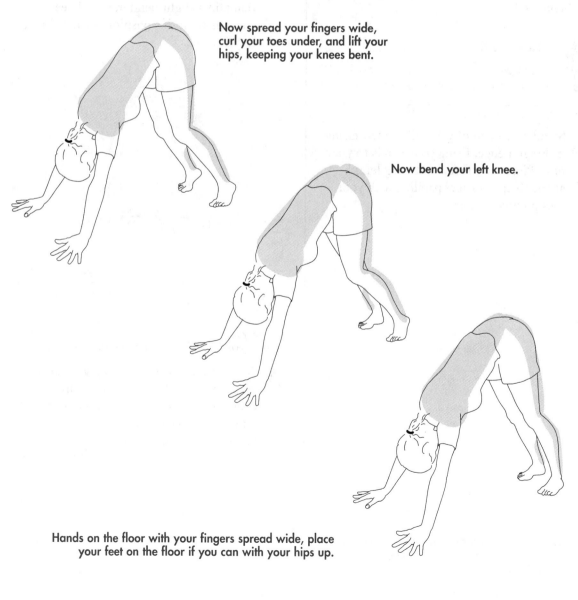

Now spread your fingers wide, curl your toes under, and lift your hips, keeping your knees bent.

Now bend your left knee.

Hands on the floor with your fingers spread wide, place your feet on the floor if you can with your hips up.

## Leap Frog

Leap Frog strengthens and stretches your spine and inner and back legs. It also relieves pressure and tension in the abdominal and pelvic area. With this stretch, you'll find fast relief from the mild backache that often arises during this time of the month. And to top it off, this stretch calms your brain and frazzled nerves that go hand in hand with PMS.

You'll need a sticky mat for this stretch. (See Appendix C for information on where you can purchase one.)

**Flex Alert!** _____

Don't practice Leap Frog if your back or hips are injured or inflamed.

1. Stand at the end of your sticky mat, facing its longest edge. Bring your hands to your hips. Place your feet about a leg length apart. Keep your feet parallel, with your toes pointed forward.

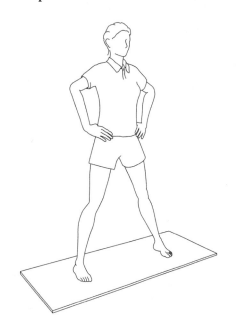

Stand on your sticky mat facing the longest edge, with your hands on your hips, your feet parallel and a leg length apart, and your toes pointed forward.

2. Inhale deeply into your chest as your raise your arms over your head. Then exhale as you bend your torso forward from your hip joints and place your hands on the mat beneath your shoulders. Repeat these movements two more times, making sure you raise your arms to your ears first before you lift up.

3. Hold the forward bend with your hands on the mat beneath your shoulders. Slide your legs wide enough apart so you can place the crown of your head on the mat. Maintain a slight bend in your knees as you remain in this position for four long, deep breaths.

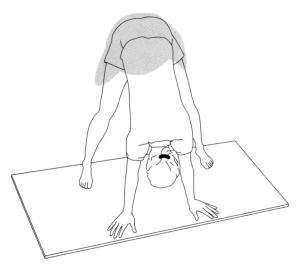

Bend your torso forward from your hip joints with your hands on the mat beneath your shoulders.

4. To release the stretch, sweep your arms up toward the sky and inhale to lift your torso. Exhale as you lower your arms to your sides and then place your feet together. Stand and rest for a few moments. Notice the effects of the stretch.

## Reclining Number 4 Stretch

The Reclining Number 4 Stretch is essentially the same routine you found in the "Hip Openers" section of Chapter 4; the only difference is that here you practice it lying on your back. It relieves symptoms associated with PMS, calms your nervous system, increases the flow of oxygenated blood to your reproductive organs, and encourages deep relaxation.

**Flex Alert!**

Omit this stretch from your routine if you suffer from sciatica or chronic back pain.

1. Lie on your back with your legs extended. Place the sole of your right foot on your left inner thigh. Your legs should be in the shape of the numeral 4. Rest your arms at your sides.

2. Hold the stretch for four deep breaths. As you inhale, feel your belly rise into your fingertips. As you exhale, feel your belly fall. Relax all your muscles, especially your inner thigh and hips.

3. Repeat steps 1 and 2 on the other side of your body. Notice if you feel any difference on this side.

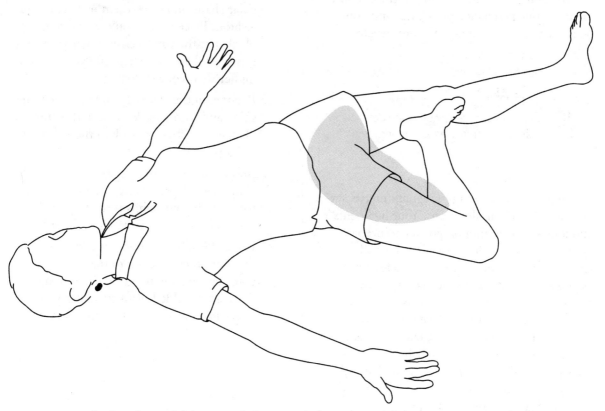

Lie on your back with your left leg extended, your right foot on your left thigh, and your legs in the shape of the numeral 4.

# Pregnancy

Staying active during your pregnancy is essential. Moving your body and stretching can help you manage your body's shifting center of gravity and assist you in sailing through your labor, delivery, and postpartum recovery with ease. Flexibility is an important way to help your muscles handle the postural adjustments your body is experiencing.

You'll enjoy stretching throughout your pregnancy as a way of releasing muscle tension so you can unwind. In addition, you may prevent injuries and increase your level of coordination and range of motion. Attending to your body helps you keep a watchful eye on how you're feeling, allowing for an effortless adjustment as your pregnancy progresses and your body adjusts to accommodate your developing baby.

**Flex Alert!**

Consult your health-care provider before you start your pregnancy stretching program.

Stretching while you're pregnant merits several important considerations. Your ligaments and joints relax during pregnancy to prepare your body for the birth of your baby, so be careful not to go beyond your muscle's limits as you stretch. Warm up by taking a shower or a walk, and watch your balance as you stretch. Never stretch in a supine (face up, on your back) position after your first trimester, as you may restrict blood flow to your baby. Keep your joints relaxed as you stretch, and always stop your routine if you experience pain, shortness of breath, nausea, or dizziness.

# Reclining Frog

Reclining Frog increases hip flexibility and stretches your inner thigh muscles. You may practice it at any stage in your pregnancy. It's a great position to hold during labor.

**S-t-r-e-t-c-h It Out**

For Reclining Frog, you'll need to gather at least four blankets and a small pillow or folded blanket for your head. You may also want to have a few extra blankets to place under your knees to support your legs and hips.

1. Fold your blankets lengthwise in a rectangular shape and stack them in a stair-step fashion. Place a small pillow or folded blanket at the top to ensure that your head is higher than your chest and your chest is higher than your abdomen.

2. Recline on the stacked blankets with your spine and whole back supported by the blankets. Rest your head on the pillow at the top.

3. Allow your arms to stretch out to the sides about a 45-degree angle away from your torso, with your palms turned upward. Alternately, rest your hands on your belly.

4. Bring the soles of your feet together and let your knees rest out to the sides. Keep your legs in a diamond shape. You may place a few folded blankets under your knees to support your legs and hips.

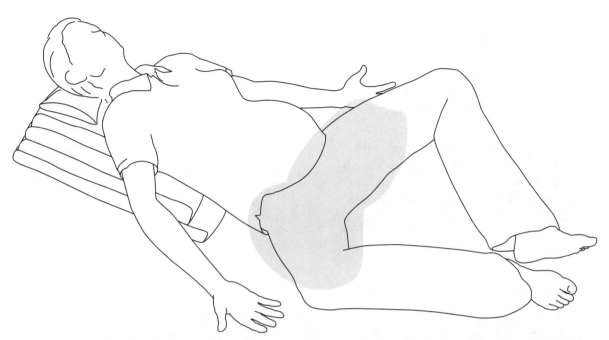

Lie on your back on four blankets placed in a stair-step fashion. Rest your head on a pillow at the top, extend your arms out about 45 degrees away from your torso with your palms up, and splay your knees out to the sides.

**Flex Alert!**

It's normal for your hips to become more flexible when your hormones change as you prepare to give birth. Even if you don't feel that you're straining your muscles, place blankets beneath your knees for added support if you're planning to stay in the stretch more than 5 minutes or if you feel any pulling or pinching at your hip joints.

5. Hold this position for at least 5 minutes. You may remain here as long as you wish, perhaps stretching for 20 or 30 minutes if you feel comfortable. Take long, slow, deep, relaxing breaths with your eyes closed.

## Modified Twist

Although deep twists aren't normally recommended for pregnant women, here's a safe way to keep your spine supple and aligned throughout your pregnancy. This twist emanates from the chest and shoulders. Your body is supported by pillows and blankets so you can relax overworked back muscles and hips. You'll also release tension and stress so you can benefit from restful sleep.

**S-t-r-e-t-c-h It Out**

Gather a large pillow for your head, neck, and shoulders, and four blankets or two large pillows to place between your legs for the Modified Twist.

1. Lie on your right side, using the pillows and blankets to support your head and neck. Bend your knees so they're stacked on top of each other. Place two folded blankets between your legs, keeping your knees aligned with your hips to prevent lower back strain.

2. Rest your arms at shoulder level, with your left and right shoulders stacked on top of one another. Rest your hands palm on palm. Take a few long, deep breaths to unwind.

3. Inhale as you lift your left arm up and back toward the floor behind you. Turn your head and neck left as you twist from your shoulders. Exhale as you return to the starting position and place your left palm on top of your right palm.

4. Repeat step 3 three more times, and then hold the position for three deep breaths.

5. Repeat the twist on your left side.

Lie on your right side with a pillow or blanket to support your head and neck, your knees bent and stacked on top of each other with two folded blankets between your legs. Keep your knees in line with your hips, your arms at shoulder level, your left and right shoulders stacked, and your hands resting palm on palm.

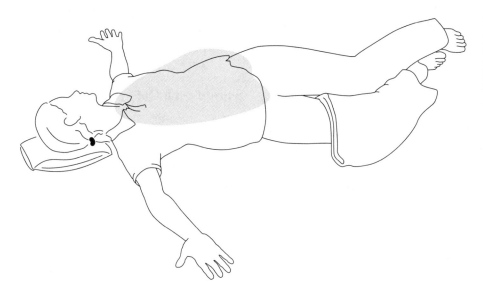

Place your left arm up and back toward the floor behind you with your head and neck turned left, twisting from your shoulders.

## Right Angle at Wall

Right Angle at Wall is beneficial in the third trimester, when the heaviness of the uterus causes your lower-back muscles to contract. This stretch relieves lower-back tension and releases tight hamstrings and calf muscles.

1. Stand facing a wall. Extend your arms straight out from your shoulders, with your hands shoulder-width apart on the wall. Keep your feet parallel and even with your hips. Stretch your toes.

2. Step back until your arms and back are parallel to the floor. Tighten your front thigh muscles, push the wall firmly, lift your kneecaps, and extend your hips away from the wall. Keep your head in line with your arms, and fully stretch your shoulders. Feel your spine and the sides of your body lengthen. Hold the stretch four deep breaths or until your back feels stretched. Keep your eyes open. Lengthen your torso with each exhale.

3. Walk your feet toward the wall as your hands climb up the wall. Then relax your arms at your sides. Pause to regulate your blood pressure.

Stand facing a wall with your arms straight out from your shoulders, your hands shoulder-width apart on the wall, and your feet parallel and hip-width apart.

## Partner Squat

Squatting is a key stretch to practice throughout your pregnancy. You'll open your pelvis and become accustomed to the most natural position for giving birth. Regular squatting increases the mobility of your pelvic and hip joints, bringing your pelvis into the proper position in relation to your spine. Muscles in your back, buttocks, hips, and pelvic floor elongate and loosen. You'll also increase circulation in your pelvic area. Practicing the squat with a partner is fun, too.

**Flex Alert!**

Do not squat if your baby is in the breech position after 34 weeks, if you've had a cervical stitch, or if you have hemorrhoids or varicose veins.

1. Stand facing your partner with your feet about a foot and a half apart, toes turned out a little.

2. Grasp each other's wrists, and move to a distance far enough away from each other so your arms are straight.

3. Inhale and then squat as you slowly exhale, adjusting your position as needed to support each other as you move. Move your knees directly over your feet, and keep your arms taut. Lean back a little to create enough tension to support each other.

4. Hold the squat for three deep breaths and then inhale slowly as you return to a standing position.

5. Repeat steps 3 and 4 two more times.

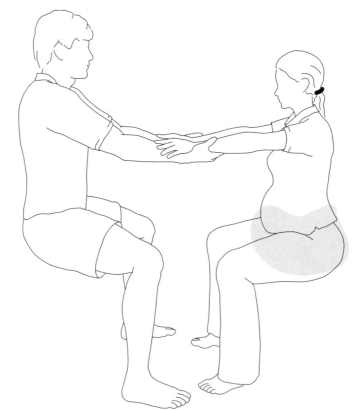

Squat with a partner, holding each other's wrists, with your arms straight, your hips close to the floor, and your knees pointed in same direction as your toes.

## Meditative Stretch

The Meditative Stretch safely and gently stretches your back, relieving lower-back tension. You may practice this stretch throughout your pregnancy as a form of conscious relaxation.

1. Kneel on a blanket or mat and inhale deeply. Slowly bring your hips back toward your heels. Then, as you exhale, bend at your hips and stretch your torso backward between your legs. Widen your heels so your belly rests between your thighs. Rest your forehead on a mat or pillow or on your folded forearms. Alternately, place your arms beside your legs for deeper relaxation.

2. Take long, deep breaths, consciously relaxing your spine and chest as you release tense muscles with each exhale. Hold the stretch for six breaths or until your whole body feels calm.

 **S-t-r-e-t-c-h It Out**

Have your partner place his or her palms on your sacrum and gently press down and back toward your feet to gently massage and release tension in your lower back.

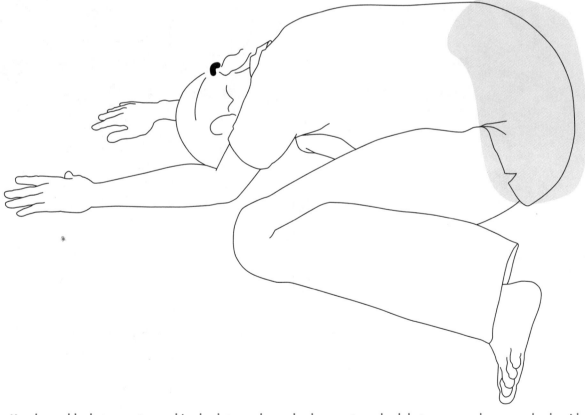

Kneel on a blanket or mat, your hips back toward your heels, your torso back between your legs, your heels widened, your belly resting between your thighs, your forehead resting on a mat or pillow, and your arms straight forward.

# Ankle Rolls

You know your body retains a higher volume of fluid when you're pregnant. Ankle Rolls relieve swelling in your feet and ankle joints, especially common in the third trimester. The stretch's circular motion helps circulate the extra fluid in your body out of your joints. Ankle Rolls are similar to Ankle Circles, found in Chapter 4.

1. Sit with your legs outstretched on a mat or blanket. Place the palms of your hands on the floor out to the sides and just behind your buttocks. Point your fingers away from your hips. Lean back slightly, using your arms as support. Keep your elbows bent slightly; your feet slightly apart; and your back, neck, and head straight.

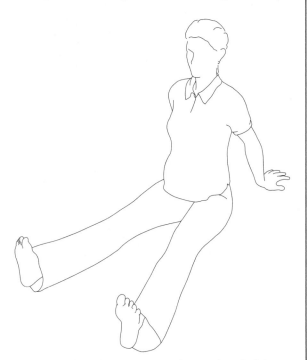

Sit with your legs outstretched, your feet slightly apart, your hands somewhat behind your buttocks, and lean back.

2. Keep your legs separated but straight. Lift your left leg a few inches from the floor. Rotate your left foot clockwise 10 times and then counterclockwise 10 times. Inhale as you move your foot up, and exhale as you move it down. Pay close attention to the circling motion, closing your eyes to avoid distraction. Notice the range of motion in each ankle as you move.

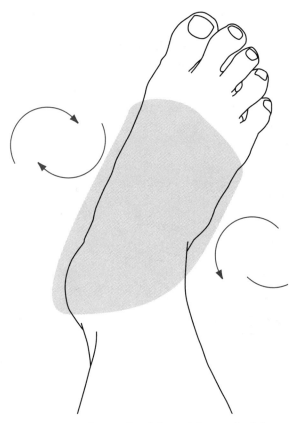

Rotate your foot to the right and then to the left.

3. Repeat step 2 with your right foot.

4. Bring both feet together, resting your heels on the mat, and rotate them at the same time clockwise 10 times and then counterclockwise 10 times.

5. Finally, separate your feet and rotate them 10 times in one direction and then 10 times in the opposite direction.

# Menopause

Every woman has her own unique experience as she moves through menopause. Some women don't suffer from any symptoms, while others endure anxiety, fatigue, backaches, headaches, insomnia, anger, sadness, and hot flashes. Each stretch in this section targets specific symptoms, so allow your symptoms to guide your stretching practice.

The time you take to stretch your way out of uncomfortable physical or emotional sensations is a gift to yourself. So have fun and enjoy experimenting with stretching—it's a great activity to address your needs during one of life's major transitions.

**S-t-r-e-t-c-h It Out**

Be sure you use envelope breathing throughout each stretch. It ensures that the benefits of each stretch take place in your body.

## Back Arch

The Back Arch relieves menopausal symptoms such as anxiety, fatigue, backaches, headaches, and insomnia. This calming stretch releases stress; rejuvenates tired legs; and stretches your chest, neck, and spine. Chest expansion helps you breathe more deeply and lifts your spirits. You also stimulate your abdominal organs to improve digestion.

1. Lie on your back on the floor or mat. Bend your knees. Keep your feet parallel and placed even with and a comfortable distance from your hips. Rest your arms by your sides, your palms down.

2. Inhale deeply and, as you exhale, press into your feet and your arms, lifting your buttocks off the floor. Don't let your knees splay out to the sides. Inhale with your hips lifted, and exhale as you lower your hips.

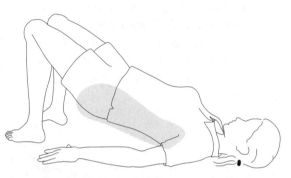

Lie on your back on the floor or mat with your knees bent and your feet hip-width apart and parallel, a comfortable distance away from your hips. Rest your arms by your sides with your palms down and your hips lifted.

3. Repeat step 2 three more times. Then hold the stretch with your hips lifted for four long, deep breaths.

4. Lower your hips as you exhale, and relax your arms and back. Rest for a few moments and enjoy the results.

# Knee Press

Perhaps you remember the Knee Press from Chapters 8 and 9. With this relaxing stretch, you release the anxiety, worry, and frazzled nerves that may accompany menopause. Practicing long, smooth exhales helps calm your mind and drive your energy downward to release pent-up feelings of anger or sadness. Knee Press also releases toxins and stretches your lower back and hips to let you unwind.

1. Lie on your back on a comfortable surface (not your bed). Take a deep breath in and then draw one knee toward your chest as you exhale. Inhale again, and with the next exhale, draw your other knee toward your chest. Place your hands lightly on each knee. Tuck your chin toward your chest, but keep your head on the floor.

2. Move your thighs away from your heart as you breathe in, straightening your arms. Keep your hands on your knees. Move your thighs toward your chest, bending your elbows as you exhale. Do not pull or force your legs toward your chest. Practice these movements eight times.

**Flex Alert!** _____

Do not practice step 3 if you have had recent abdominal surgery or if you experience pain after trying one repetition.

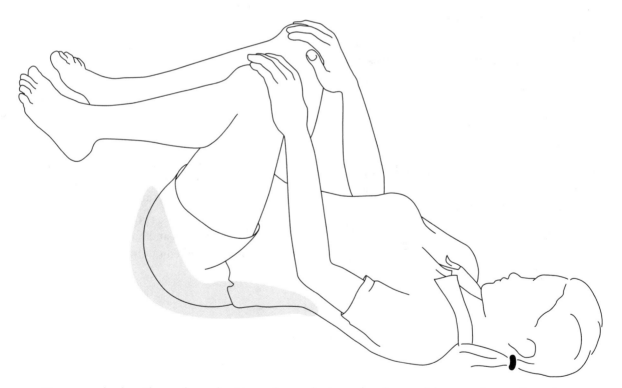

Lie on your back, with your knees bent toward your chest, one hand on each knee, and your elbows bent.

3. With your head resting on the floor, grasp your arms around your knees, forming a ball. Hold on to your hand, wrist, or forearm as you draw your knees toward your chest. Rest your head on the floor. Take one deep, full breath in this position. Inhale, and as you exhale, bring your nose toward your knees, engaging your abdominal muscles as you move.

4. Lower your upper back to the floor and relax your shoulders as you inhale. Repeat these movements two more times, then rest with your hands on your knees for a few moments.

Lie on your back, with your knees bent, your arms wrapped around your legs, your head on the floor, and curl your nose up to your knees.

Lie on your back, with your knees bent toward your chest, one hand on each knee, and your arms straight.

# Heels Over Head Stretch

You might also recall the Heels Over Head Stretch from Chapters 6 and 8. It helps relieve tired and cramped legs and feet by gently stretching the back of your legs, your front torso, and the back of your neck. It also calms your mind and balances your hormones to prevent and treat symptoms of menopause such as hot flashes, insomnia, sadness, and anxiety.

1. Lie on your right side, close to a wall, with your knees bent toward your chest. Scoot your hips so your feet and buttocks touch the wall.

2. Roll to the left, swinging your legs up the wall. Open your arms from your shoulders out to the sides, palms up. If you feel tension in the backs of your legs, turn your legs slightly in and release any tightness in your knees.

**Flex Alert!**

Be sure your buttocks touch the wall. You may bend your knees slightly if you feel any pulling sensations in the backs of your legs.

3. Relax into the stretch and breathe deeply, holding the position at least 5 minutes. Your breathing becomes slow and deep as you hold the stretch, relieving stress and relaxing muscles in your forehead, eyes, jaw, and tongue.

4. Come out of the stretch, retracing the steps you took to move into it. Bend your knees, roll to your side, and use your strong arms to move to your hands and knees. Place one foot on the floor, knee bent, and hold on to a chair or the wall for support as you raise your body to standing.

**Lie on your right side, your knees bent, your feet and buttocks touching the wall.**

**Lie on your back with your legs up the wall and your arms out to the sides.**

## J Stretch

This powerful stretch helps relieve symptoms of menopause and also soothes your brain; reduces stress and fatigue; and stretches your back, shoulders, and spine. You need a chair or small bench for this stretch.

**Flex Alert!** _____

Do not practice the J Stretch during menstruation or if your back or neck is sore or injured.

1. Practice the J Stretch on a rug, or place a mat or folded blanket, at least the size of your torso, on the floor. Position your chair at the top of the soft surface so when you move your legs back over your head, you can rest them on the chair.

2. Lie flat on your back on the soft surface, your arms by your sides, your palms face down. Inhale deeply and then, as you exhale, press your hands and arms into the floor to assist you as you raise your legs, lifting your trunk and swinging your legs back behind your head so they rest on the chair.

3. Place your hands on your back, and support your back with your upper arms and elbows placed firmly on the ground. Allow your upper back to relax as much as possible to bring your legs as far over onto the chair as you comfortably can—eventually, the chair should support your thighs. Your body should look like the letter *J*. Hold the stretch at least four long breaths or longer.

4. To release the stretch, use your arms as support while you very slowly lower your entire spine to a lying position. Rest for a few breaths. Notice how the stretch has affected your body and mind.

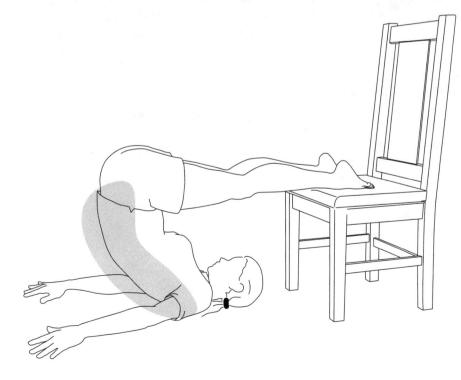

**Lie on your back with your legs back over your head and resting on a chair. Your body should look like the letter J.**

# Mindful Stretching for Stress Relief

Stress is a natural condition of our complex and demanding lives in the twenty-first century. Our bodies remain in a state of continuous low-level stress. You may experience stress as exhaustion, loss of energy, and impaired awareness and creativity. Pressures at work, family obligations, and social and legal customs all create demands on your body, creating tension, irritability, and fatigue—and possibly more serious health issues down the road.

Have you ever caught yourself tensing your shoulders or clenching your jaw? Muscle tension builds as you work through challenging days. Faced with difficult circumstances, your body reacts with a series of physical responses that rally internal forces, preparing you to take action. Twenty thousand years ago, when danger approached, we either attacked in self-defense or fled the scene. Hans Selye, the father of stress studies, named this the "fight or flight" syndrome. For early man, whose stress was primarily physical in nature, the choice was relatively one or the other, and often easy to make.

Nowadays, however, we experience more complex mental and emotional types of stress. Nevertheless, our bodies still respond with the same chemical reactions as early man. This reaction can lead to *burnout*, which plagues contemporary society. We suffer from a host of stress-related conditions such as insomnia, digestive disorders, and immune system deficiencies. Headaches, backaches, and major illnesses such as heart disease, cancer, and strokes are also considered stress-related illnesses.

**Flexicon**

The result of living in a state of continuous stress, **burnout** is long-term physical and emotional exhaustion, sometimes leading to a diminished interest in life.

Stress relief through regular stretching helps you be more resourceful and provides you a subtle way to let go as you relax tight muscles that often accompany stress. Each stretch provides a releasing sensation, invigorating yet relaxing. Your muscles rest so you can breathe more easily. Your can lower your heart rate and blood pressure as all your internal systems recharge, allowing your body to heal. You may find your attention more focused and your emotions and moods stabilized. Stretching helps you clear your mind as you create a more stable, creative, and blissful state of mind.

## Z Stretch

Also found in Chapter 8, the Z Stretch helps release tension from your spinal column and muscles. Stress is often stored in the shoulders and hips; the Z Stretch gently stretches those areas as well as your lower back.

**S-t-r-e-t-c-h It Out**

Use a firm, folded blanket under your knees to protect these precious parts of your body.

1. Kneel on a blanket or rug with your knees placed directly beneath your hips and your shoulders positioned directly above your wrists. Spread your fingers wide. Relax your shoulders. Inhale deeply into your chest, lifting your chin slightly at the top of the breath.

2. As you exhale, bring your chin toward your chest, your chest toward your thighs, and your hips toward your heels, moving into a crouching position like the letter Z.

3. Repeat steps 1 and 2 seven more times, and then rest in the Z position for four deep breaths.

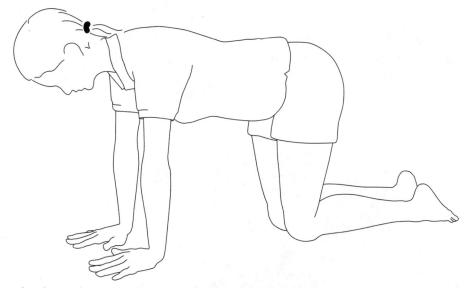

Kneel with your knees beneath your hips, your shoulders positioned directly above your wrists, and your fingers spread.

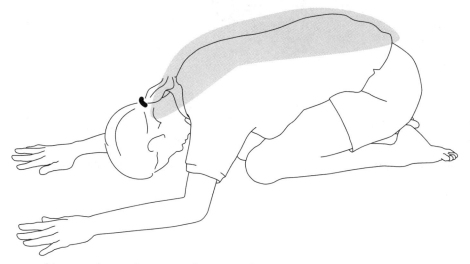

Bring your chin toward your chest, your chest toward your thighs, and your hips toward your heels.

## Reclining Diamond

This forward bend helps release stress so you can sleep. Reclining Diamond is a perfect stretch for your inner-thigh muscles and the nerve fibers in your groin. It loosens joints in your lower body, massages your internal organs, and strengthens your back and spine. Rest easy with this amazing stretch.

1. Lie on a comfortable surface. Bring the soles of your feet together, with your heels a comfortable distance away from your groin. Your legs should be in the shape of a diamond.

2. Hold this position for four long, smooth breaths, or even longer if you wish. Relax and let gravity do the work. Notice where you feel the stretch in your body.

**A Stretch in Time ...**

Work the Reclining Diamond stretch into your evening routine, moving into the stretch while you watch television or when you climb into bed, to ensure restful sleep.

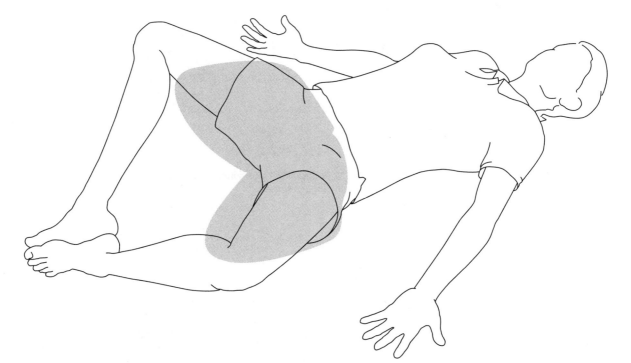

**Lie with your knees bent, the soles of your feet together, and your legs in a diamond shape.**

Lie on your back with your arms stretched out from your shoulders in a T position, the sole of your right foot on top of your right knee, your torso twisted to the left, and your right knee moving toward your left hand.

## Reclining Twist

Found in the "Golf and Tennis" section of Chapter 9, this twist wrings the tension and stress out of your spinal column, releases toxins, and improves circulation of blood and oxygen to your muscles. Say good-bye to the shoulder and neck stiffness that creeps up during a stressful day.

**Flex Alert!**

Do not practice the Reclining Twist if your back is sore or injured. Never force or strain.

1. Lie on your back with your arms stretched out from your shoulders in a *T* position. Scoot your hips to the right a few inches.
2. Place the sole of your right foot lightly on top of your right knee. Inhale deeply into your chest.
3. Twist your torso to the left, and as you exhale, bring your right knee toward your left hand and turn your head to the right.
4. Unwind your torso back to the starting position as you inhale.
5. Repeat steps 3 and 4 three more times. Then hold the twist for four deep breaths.
6. Repeat the twist on the other side of your body.

## The Least You Need to Know

◆ Set a date with yourself to practice the A Frame, Leap Frog, and Reclining Number 4 stretches to ward off PMS.

◆ Stretching is a safe activity to enjoy throughout your pregnancy and helps you meet the joys and challenges that motherhood brings to your life.

◆ If you've decided to step through menopause without hormone replacement therapy, you're not alone. Make stretching a tool to help manage this important transition.

◆ Stress is an integral part of your life. You cannot escape stress, but you can manage it by stretching—it's your best insurance to prevent stress-related disease.

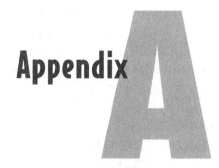

**Appendix A**

# Glossary

**aerobic exercise**   Any type of exercise, typically performed at moderate levels of intensity for extended periods of time, that maintains an increased heart rate.

**alignment**   The proper placement of the bones so the muscles do less work.

**arthritis**   A group of conditions in which damage has been caused to the joints of the body.

**asymmetrical**   Having no balance or symmetry.

**balance**   Equilibrium, which maintains physical balance in humans and animals.

**blocks**   Small wooden, cork, or foam rectangles that may be used to support your body and provide stability while stretching.

**bolster**   A long, narrow pillow or cushion.

**burnout**   The result of living in a state of continuous stress, burnout is long-term physical and emotional exhaustion, sometimes leading to a diminished interest in life.

**cartilage**   A type of dense connective tissue that provides smooth surfaces for the smooth movement of bones.

**circulation**   The movement of blood through bodily vessels as a result of the heart's pumping action.

**colon**   The section of the large intestine extending from the cecum to the rectum. Its primary purpose is to extract water from feces.

**contract**   To reduce in size by or as if by being drawn together.

**contraindication**   A factor that renders the administration of a drug or the carrying out of a procedure inadvisable.

**crown**   The top of the head.

**dynamic stretching**   Moving your body in and out of a stretch, allowing your body to adjust to a stretch before you hold it.

**edge**   A place of neither too much nor too little stretch. This place marks the healthy limit of your body's flexibility, and the place where your mind is naturally focused.

**elasticity**   The condition or property of being flexible.

**elongate**   To lengthen.

**envelope breathing**   To "envelop" your movements with breath. Start to breathe before you move, and end your movement with breath to spare. The flow of your breath naturally inspires and initiates the movement.

**expand**   To increase the size, volume, quantity, or scope of; to enlarge.

**fascia**   Specialized connective tissue surrounding muscles, bones, and joints that provides your body support, protection, and structure.

**fatigue**   Physical or mental weariness resulting from exertion.

**flat back**   Means that your back is as flat as a table. With time and practice, you'll be able to feel the difference between a flat back and a rounded back. Try to stretch by a mirror to check for a flat back.

**flexibility**   The ability of your muscles, tendons, and ligaments to stretch, which allows your joints to have a larger range of movement. This component is important to avoid injuries during leisure activities.

**frozen shoulder** (*adhesive capsulitis*)   A condition in which the shoulder capsule, the connective tissue surrounding your shoulder joint, becomes irritated and inflexible, causing severe loss of mobility in your shoulder.

**herniated**   To protrude through an abnormal bodily opening.

**hip flexors**   A set of muscles found in your pelvis that bend your hips and rotate your lower spine.

**hip rotators**   A group of six muscles that help your hips rotate either inward or outward.

**imbalance**   A state of loss of equilibrium attributable to an unstable situation in which some forces outweigh others (as may occur in cases of inner ear disease).

**immobile**   Not capable of movement or of being moved.

**immune system**   A bodily system (including the thymus and bone marrow and lymphoid tissues) that protects the body from foreign substances and pathogenic organisms by producing the immune response.

**insomnia**   A chronic inability to fall asleep or remain asleep for an adequate length of time.

**intercostal muscles**   Several groups of muscles that run between the ribs and help form and move the chest wall.

**intervertebral**   Located between vertebrae.

**joint**   The location where two bones make contact.

**joint capsules**   Bags of connective tissue that secrete and hold the synovial fluid that lubricates the joint.

**lactic acid**   A chemical byproduct that causes muscles to ache when exercised.

**ligaments**   Short bands of tough connective tissue that connect bones to other bones to form a joint.

**meniscus**   A crescent-shape cartilage disc cushioning the end of a bone where it meets another bone in a joint, especially in the knee.

**musculoskeletal**   Relates to your skeleton, joints, muscles, and tendons.

**ocular**   Related to the eyes.

**osteoarthritis**   A condition in which joints become inflamed and painful, caused by the degeneration of the cartilage that protects and acts as a cushion inside your joints.

**pelvis**   A basin-shape structure of the vertebrate skeleton, composed of the bones on the sides, the pubis in front, and the sacrum and coccyx behind, that rests on the lower limbs and supports the spinal column.

**piriformis muscle**   A muscle that extends from the side of the sacrum to the top of the thigh bone at the hip joint, passing over the sciatic nerve.

**posture**   A position of the body or of body parts; placing the body in a particular position.

**prone**   Lying with the front or face downward.

**proprioception**   Your natural sense of the position of the parts of your body in relation to each other.

**proprioceptive neuromuscular facilitation (PNF)**   A technique of alternating stretching and contracting repeatedly to stretch a bit farther each time.

**psoas muscles**   Muscles located on each side of your back. Chronically tight in most people, they originate at the spine around the bottom of the rib cage and run down to the pelvis and thigh bone.

**range of motion**   The measurement of the achievable distance between the flexed position and the extended position of a particular joint or muscle group.

**rehabilitative**   To restore to good health or useful life, as through therapy and education.

**relaxation**   The act of relaxing or the state of being relaxed.

**repetitive**   Given to or characterized by repeating the same movement or action.

**resistance**   A force that tends to oppose or retard motion.

**restorative**   Something that replenishes.

**sacrum**   A flat, triangular bone at the base of your spine.

**static stretching**   When you place your body in a stretch and hold the stretch for a number of breaths.

**sternum**   Commonly called the "breastbone," your sternum is a long, flat bone in the center of your chest. Connected to your ribs with cartilage, the sternum protects your lungs and heart.

**strength**   The ability of a person or animal to exert force on physical objects using muscles.

**stress**   The sum of physical and mental responses to an unacceptable disparity between real or imagined personal experience and personal expectations.

**stretching**   The activity of contracting and releasing muscles to lengthen, strengthen, and lubricate them.

**structural misalignment**   When the body's natural posture is altered due to gravity, the stress of daily activities, or physical injuries.

**supine**   Lying on your back, or face up.

**supple**   Pliant or flexible.

**symmetrical**   Having similarity in size, shape, and relative position of corresponding parts.

**synovial fluid**   A thin, stringy liquid found in joint cavities that reduces friction between cartilage and other tissues. Synovial fluid lubricates and cushions joints during movement.

**temporal bones**   Bones found at the sides and base of your skull.

**temporomandibular joint disorder (TMJD)**   A variety of conditions that cause pain and discomfort in the temporomandibular joint where your lower jawbone joins the temporal bone of your skull.

**tendons**   Tough bands of fibrous tissues that connect muscle to bone.

**tension**   The act or process of stretching something tight.

**toxin**   A poisonous substance, especially a protein, produced by living cells or organisms that's capable of causing disease when introduced into the body tissues. Often a toxin is also capable of inducing neutralizing antibodies or antitoxins.

**vertebra**   One of the bony segments of the spinal column.

**vitality**   An energetic style.

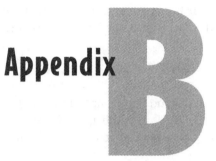

# Program Appendix

Streamline your stretching program with these customized routines. These 10-, 20-, or 30-minute routines provide you with essential stretches designed to maximize your time and effort. No need to mix and match, just follow these simple instructions to add energy and flexibility into your life.

# 10-Minute Stretch Routine

This 10-minute routine opens your chest so you can breathe deeper. A side stretch and twist targets your precious spine. Practice this program every morning to feel alive and move freely throughout the day, or use this 10-minute sequence to unwind after a long day.

## Receiving Stretch (Chapter 5)

1. Stand with your arms at your sides, your feet hip-width apart. Close your eyes for a moment, if you feel steady, and relax.

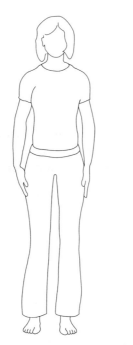

**Start the Receiving Stretch standing with your arms at your sides and your feet hip-width apart.**

2. S-t-r-e-t-c-h your arms out to your sides and up over your head, inhaling as you move.

3. Look up at your palms as they come together. Relax your shoulders. Pause.

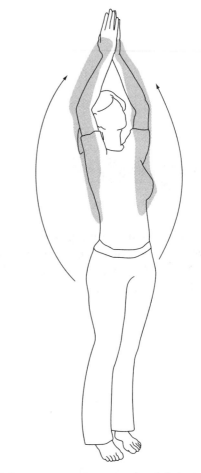

**Raise your arms over your head, bringing your palms together like in a prayer, and look up.**

4. Exhale. Allow your arms to float back down to your sides. Pause.

5. Repeat these movements two more times.

# Gentle Side Stretch (Chapter 5)

1. Start standing with your feet hip-width apart, arms by your sides.

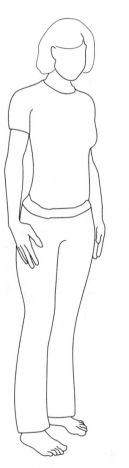

**Begin by standing with your feet hip-width apart and your arms by your sides.**

2. Sweep your left arm up by your ear, palm turned in, inhaling as you go. S-t-r-e-t-c-h.

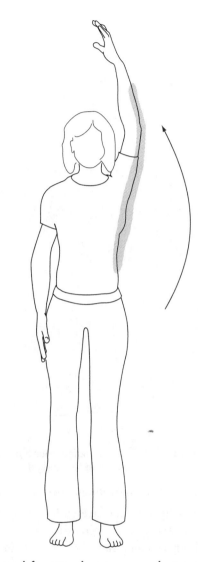

**Stretch your left arm up by your ear, palm turned in, while your right arm rests by your side.**

3. Bend, gliding your hips to the left and your torso to the right, as you exhale. Gaze forward.

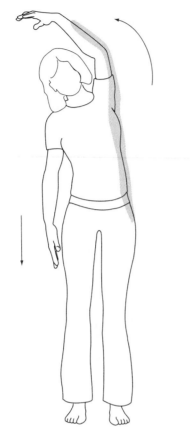

**Stretch your left side by bending your hips to the left and your torso to the right.**

4. Repeat the movements two more times.

5. Finally, hold the stretch four long inhales and exhales, engaging the core of your body as you exhale to protect your back. Do not twist, and keep your gaze forward.

6. Slowly lift your left arm and torso as you inhale. Lower your left arm to your side, exhaling as you go. Stand straight.

7. Raise your right arm up by your ear, palm turned in, inhaling as you s-t-r-e-t-c-h.

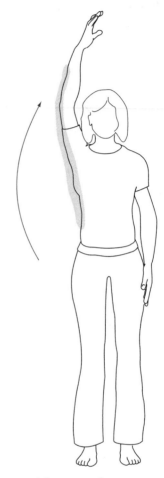

**Raise your right arm up by your ear, palm turned in, while your left arm rests by your side.**

8. Bend, gliding your hips to the right and your torso to the left, as you exhale. Look forward.

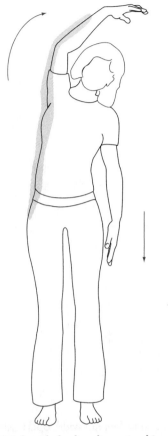

**Stretch your right side by bending your hips to the right and your torso to the left.**

9. Repeat the stretch two more times.

10. Hold the stretch for four deep breaths, moving deeper into the side stretch.

11. To release the stretch, slowly lift your right arm and torso as you inhale. Exhale, and lower your right arm to your side, to standing. Notice how each side of your body feels.

# Gentle Twist (Chapter 5)

1. Stand, feet hip-width apart, with your hands on your hips. Inhale.

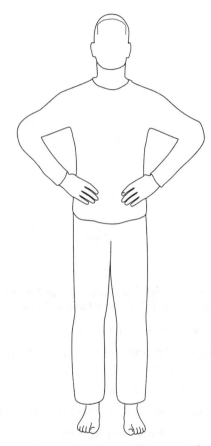

**Stand with your feet hips-width apart with your hands on your hips.**

2. Twist your torso to the right, looking over your right shoulder, exhaling as you twist. Pause to feel the twist.

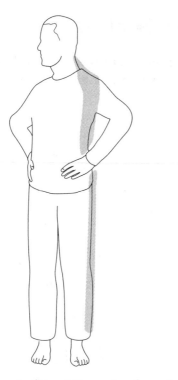

**Stand with your feet hip-width apart and your hands on your hips. Twist your torso to the right.**

3. Unwind to center as you inhale.

4. Repeat the twist as you exhale, turning a little deeper.

5. Inhale as you unwind.

6. Repeat these movements one more time.

7. Remain in the twist for four long inhales and exhales.

8. Unwind as you inhale and come back to the starting position.

9. Now twist your torso to the left, looking over your left shoulder, exhaling as you move.

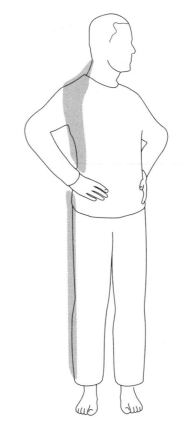

**Stand with your feet hip-width apart with your hands on your hips. Twist your torso to the left.**

10. Unwind to center as you inhale.

11. Repeat the twist as you exhale, turning a little deeper.

12. Inhale as you unwind.

13. Repeat these movements one more time.

14. Hold the twist for four long breaths.

15. Release the stretch as you breathe in.

16. Exhale. Relax your arms beside your body and feel the effects of the twist.

# 20-Minute Stretch Routine

If you have 20 minutes to spare, you can most of the bases. Begin by warming up your body as you stretch your intercostal muscles to help you breathe deeper. Move on and meet your shoulders, spine, and sides. End with the Half and Full Back stretches to target the tightest side of your body. Discover the joy of taking care of yourself. You deserve it!

## Shoulder and Chest Expander (Chapter 5)

1. Stand, feet hip-width apart, chin to chest.

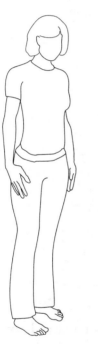

**Stand with your feet hip-width apart and your chin tucked.**

2. S-t-r-e-t-c-h your arms out to the sides and up as you inhale.

3. Interlace your fingers, press your palms up, and s-t-r-e-t-c-h.

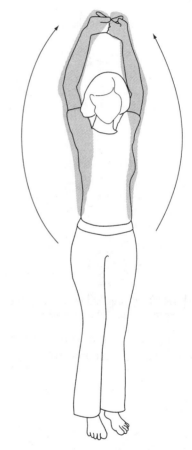

**Stand with your arms up, and interlace your fingers for an added stretch.**

4. Lean back and sweep your arms out, palms up, exhaling.

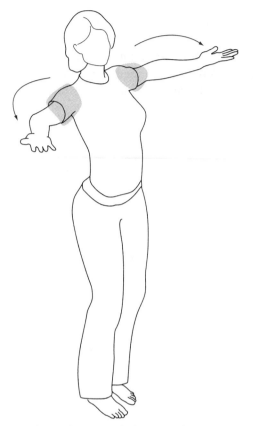

**Lean back watching your balance, and sweep your arms out and then forward.**

5. End standing straight, your arms stretched forward, your palms upward.

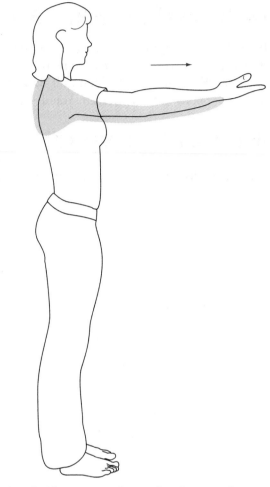

**Stand with your arms forward, palms turned up.**

6. Again, lean back and sweep your arms out, palms up, as you inhale.

7. End standing straight, your arms stretched over your head. Interlace your fingers, press your palms up, and s-t-r-e-t-c-h.

8. S-t-r-e-t-c-h your arms out to the sides and down, exhaling. Pause.

9. Practice steps 1 through 6 two more times.

# Strong Side Stretch (Chapter 5)

1. Stand with your feet and anklebones together, your chin tucked.

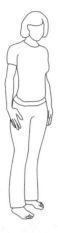

**Stand with your feet together, chin tucked, and arms to your sides.**

2. Sweep both arms out to your sides, inhaling as you stretch. Interlace your fingers, press your palms skyward, and s-t-r-e-t-c-h.

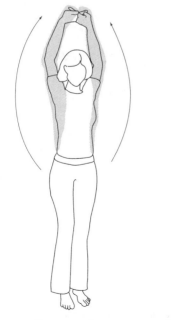

**Interlace your fingers and press your palms to the sky.**

3. Sway to the right, exhaling as you go. Feel a nice stretch up the left side of your body.

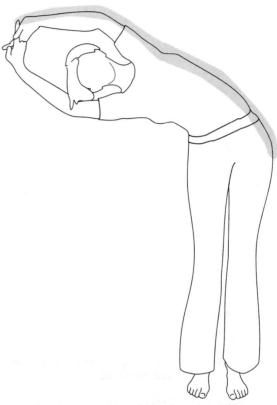

**Bend to the right with your fingers interlaced and your arms extended.**

4. Inhale back to standing.
5. S-t-r-e-t-c-h your side again as you exhale.
6. Repeat these movements one more time, stretching right.
7. Hold the stretch for four long breaths.
8. Inhale back to standing.
9. Sway your body to the left. Exhale as you s-t-r-e-t-c-h.

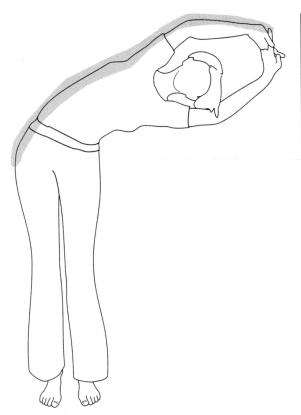

**Bend to the left with your fingers interlaced and your arms extended.**

10. Inhale back to standing.
11. Stretch your side again as you exhale.
12. Repeat the stretch one more time, then hold the stretch for four long breaths.
13. Inhale back to standing.
14. Exhale and lower both arms to your sides. Pause to feel the effects of the work.

# Strong Twist (Chapter 5)

1. Stand, feet together and chin tucked.

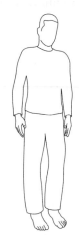

**Stand with your feet together, arms to your sides and tuck your chin.**

2. S-t-r-e-t-c-h your arms out to the sides and up over your head, inhaling as you move.

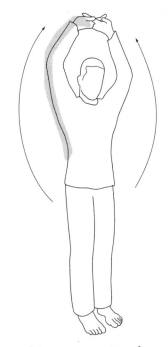

**Feel the stretch in your arms. Your fingers are interlaced and palms up.**

3. Twist your torso to the right, looking over your right shoulder, exhaling as you twist.

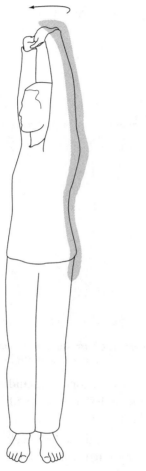

**Stand with your arms up, your fingers interlaced, your palms up. Twist your torso to the right.**

4. Inhale and release the twist.

5. Repeat the twist, exhaling as you go. Turn a little deeper this time, if you can.

6. Inhale and unwind.

7. Repeat these movements one more time.

8. Hold the twist for four breaths, lengthening your spine as you inhale. Deepen the twist as you exhale.

9. Come back to center as you inhale.

10. Exhale as you release your fingers and arms back to your sides.

11. Raise your arms out and up, interlacing your fingers at the top and inhaling as you s-t-r-e-t-c-h.

12. This time twist to the left, looking over your left shoulder, exhaling as you go.

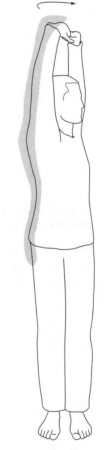

**Stand with your arms up, your fingers interlaced, and your palms up. Twist your torso to the left.**

13. Release the twist, inhaling as you move.

14. Repeat the twist as you exhale.

15. Move out of the twist as you breathe in and twist again, exhaling as you s-t-r-e-t-c-h.

16. Remain in the strong twist four long, smooth breaths.

17. Inhale back to center.

18. Lower your arms as you breathe out.

# Strong Half-Back Stretch (Chapter 5)

1. Stand with your feet and anklebones together, your chin tucked.

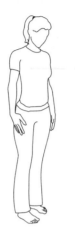

Stand with your feet together, your arms to your sides your chin tucked.

2. Sweep your arms out and up, inhaling as you go. Interlace your fingers, press your palms up, and s-t-r-e-t-c-h.

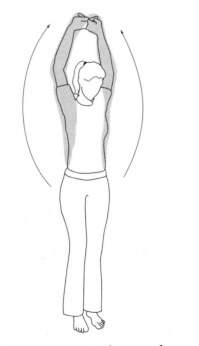

Stand with your arms up, interlace your fingers, and turn your palms up.

3. Exhale and bend halfway forward, fingers interlaced, flat back, hinging from your hips. Keep your arms by your ears and your chin to your chest.

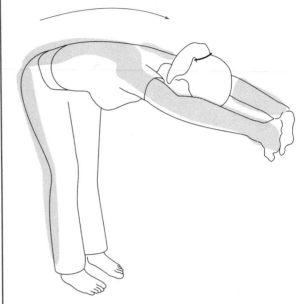

Bend forward, arms out, and fingers interlaced for a that extra-special stretch.

4. Lift your torso to standing, inhaling as you move. Exhale and bend halfway forward. Repeat these movements one more time.

5. Now hold the half back stretch for four long inhales and exhales.

6. Straighten your torso to standing. Release your arms to your sides.

# Strong Full Back Stretch (Chapter 5)

1. Stand with your feet and anklebones together, your chin tucked.

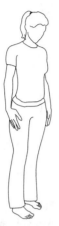

Stand with your arms to your sides, your chin to your chest.

2. S-t-r-e-t-c-h your arms out and up. Inhale. Interlace your fingers, press your palms up, and s-t-r-e-t-c-h.

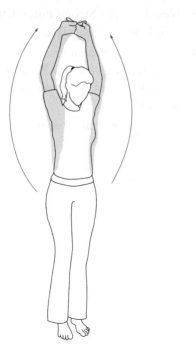

Stretch your arms up, fingers interlaced, and press your palms up. Breathe.

3. Release your fingers, and face your palms forward.

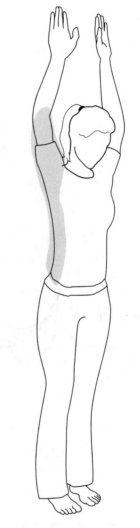

Release your fingers and allow your palms to turn forward.

4. Bend forward, hinging from the hips, exhaling as you move. Keep your back flat. Imagine that an object you want to touch is just beyond your reach. Place your hands by your feet, bending your knees, if needed.

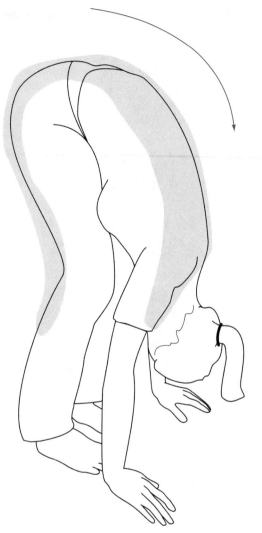

Bend forward placing your hands by your feet. It's okay to bend your knees.

5. Raise your arms to your ears, interlace your fingers, lift your torso, and s-t-r-e-t-c-h. Inhale.

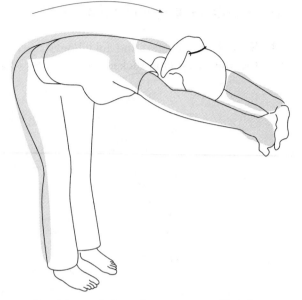

Bend forward. Extend your arms and interlace your fingers.

6. Release your fingers, face your palms forward, and dive again, exhaling as you go.

7. Repeat these movements one more time. Move with your breath.

8. Now hold the Strong Full Back Stretch four long inhales and exhales.

9. Inhale and lift your arms to your ears. Interlace your fingers. Press your palms away. Inhale as you move to a standing position.

10. Lower your arms to your sides as you exhale.

# 30-Minute Stretch Routine

Welcome, serious stretcher. You know how important it is to stretch and are willing to devote an uninterrupted 30 minutes of time to your most important asset, your body. Reap the rewards of breathing deeper and stretching the major parts of the body. You'll have more energy and enjoy checking in with yourself every day. This 30-minute routine covers all the vital stretches to insure you walk free and easy as you increase your flexibility and strength one stretch at a time.

## Shoulder and Chest Expander (Chapter 5)

1. Stand, feet hip-width apart, chin to chest.

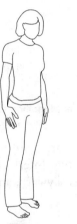

Stand with your feet hip-width apart and your chin tucked.

2. S-t-r-e-t-c-h your arms out to the sides and up as you inhale.

3. Interlace your fingers, press your palms up, and s-t-r-e-t-c-h.

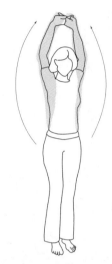

Stand with your arms up, and interlace your fingers for an added stretch.

4. Lean back and sweep your arms out, palms up, exhaling.

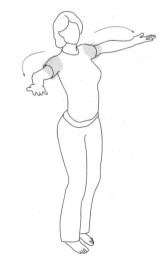

Lean back watching your balance, and sweep your arms out and then forward.

5. End standing straight, your arms stretched forward, your palms upward.

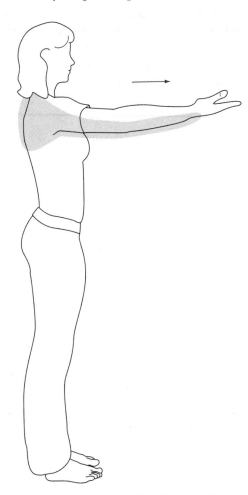

Stand with your arms forward, palms turned up.

6. Again, lean back and sweep your arms out, palms up, as you inhale.

7. End standing straight, your arms stretched over your head. Interlace your fingers, press your palms up, and s-t-r-e-t-c-h.

8. S-t-r-e-t-c-h your arms out to the sides and down, exhaling. Pause.

9. Practice steps 1 through 6 two more times.

## Strong Side Stretch (Chapter 5)

1. Stand with your feet and anklebones together, your chin tucked.

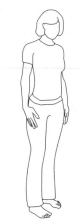

Stand with your feet together, chin tucked, and arms to your sides.

2. Sweep both arms out to your sides, inhaling as you stretch. Interlace your fingers, press your palms skyward, and s-t-r-e-t-c-h.

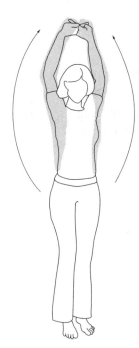

Interlace your fingers and press your palms to the sky.

3. Sway to the right, exhaling as you go. Feel a nice stretch up the left side of your body.

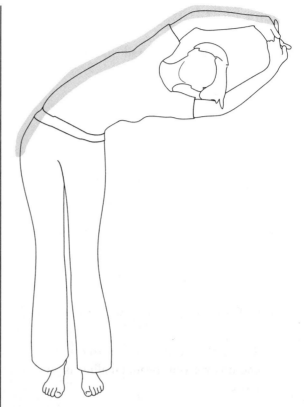

**Bend to the right with your fingers interlaced and your arms extended.**

4. Inhale back to standing.
5. S-t-r-e-t-c-h your side again as you exhale.
6. Repeat these movements one more time, stretching right.
7. Hold the stretch for four long breaths.
8. Inhale back to standing.
9. Sway your body to the left. Exhale as you s-t-r-e-t-c-h.

**Bend to the left with your fingers interlaced and your arms extended.**

10. Inhale back to standing.
11. Stretch your side again as you exhale.
12. Repeat the stretch one more time, then hold the stretch for four long breaths.
13. Inhale back to standing.
14. Exhale and lower both arms to your sides. Pause to feel the effects of the work.

## Strong Twist (Chapter 5)

1. Stand, feet together and chin tucked.

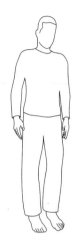

Stand with your feet together, arms to your sides and tuck your chin.

2. S-t-r-e-t-c-h your arms out to the sides and up over your head, inhaling as you move.

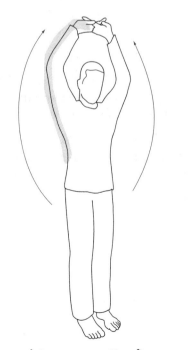

Feel the stretch in your arms. Your fingers are interlaced and palms up.

3. Twist your torso to the right, looking over your right shoulder, exhaling as you twist.

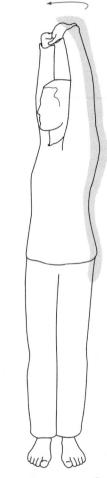

Stand with your arms up, your fingers interlaced, your palms up. Twist your torso to the right.

4. Inhale and release the twist.
5. Repeat the twist, exhaling as you go. Turn a little deeper this time, if you can.
6. Inhale and unwind.
7. Repeat these movements one more time.
8. Hold the twist for four breaths, lengthening your spine as you inhale. Deepen the twist as you exhale.

9. Come back to center as you inhale.

10. Exhale as you release your fingers and arms back to your sides.

11. Raise your arms out and up, interlacing your fingers at the top and inhaling as you s-t-r-e-t-c-h.

12. This time twist to the left, looking over your left shoulder, exhaling as you go.

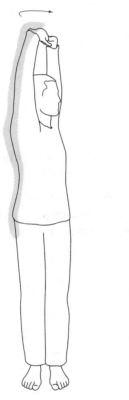

Stand with your arms up, your fingers interlaced, and your palms up. Twist your torso to the left.

13. Release the twist, inhaling as you move.

14. Repeat the twist as you exhale.

15. Move out of the twist as you breathe in and twist again, exhaling as you s-t-r-e-t-c-h.

16. Remain in the strong twist four long, smooth breaths.

17. Inhale back to center.

18. Lower your arms as you breathe out.

## Strong Half-Back Stretch (Chapter 5)

1. Stand with your feet and anklebones together, your chin tucked.

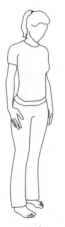

Stand with your feet together, your arms to your sides your chin tucked.

2. Sweep your arms out and up, inhaling as you go. Interlace your fingers, press your palms up, and s-t-r-e-t-c-h.

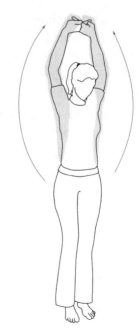

Stand with your arms up, interlace your fingers, and turn your palms up.

3. Exhale and bend halfway forward, fingers interlaced, flat back, hinging from your hips. Keep your arms by your ears and your chin to your chest.

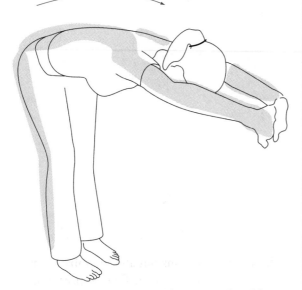

Bend forward, arms out, and fingers interlaced for a that extra-special stretch.

4. Lift your torso to standing, inhaling as you move. Exhale and bend halfway forward. Repeat these movements one more time.

5. Now hold the half back stretch for four long inhales and exhales.

6. Straighten your torso to standing. Release your arms to your sides.

## Strong Full Back Stretch (Chapter 5)

1. Stand with your feet and anklebones together, your chin tucked.

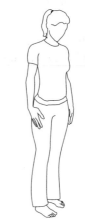

Stand with your arms to your sides, your chin to your chest.

2. S-t-r-e-t-c-h your arms out and up. Inhale. Interlace your fingers, press your palms up, and s-t-r-e-t-c-h.

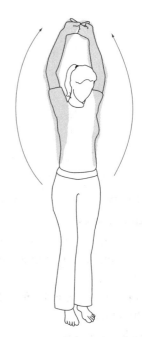

Stretch your arms up, fingers interlaced, and press your palms up. Breathe.

3. Release your fingers, and face your palms forward.

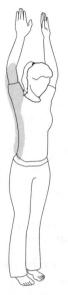

**Release your fingers and allow your palms to turn forward.**

4. Bend forward, hinging from the hips, exhaling as you move. Keep your back flat. Imagine an object you want to touch is just beyond your reach. Place your hands by your feet, bending your knees, if needed.

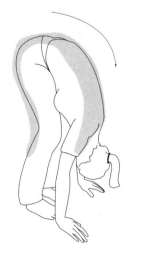

**Bend forward placing your hands by your feet. It's okay to bend your knees.**

5. Raise your arms to your ears, interlace your fingers, lift your torso, and s-t-r-e-t-c-h. Inhale.

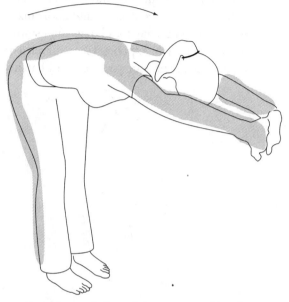

**Bend forward. Extend your arms and interlace your fingers.**

6. Release your fingers, face your palms forward, and dive again, exhaling as you go.

7. Repeat these movements one more time. Move with your breath.

8. Now hold the Strong Full Back Stretch four long inhales and exhales.

9. Inhale and lift your arms to your ears. Interlace your fingers. Press your palms away. Inhale as you move to a standing position.

10. Lower your arms to your sides as you exhale.

# Standing Hip Flexor Stretch (Chapter 4)

1. Stand steadily on a firm surface, with your feet even with your hips and your arms at your sides. Practice balance and coordination. Spreading your toes helps you establish a firm base of support. Gaze forward at one object to enhance your sense of balance.

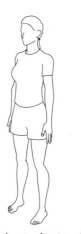

**Stand steadily to begin the Standing Hip Flexor Stretch, your feet hip-width apart and your arms at your sides.**

2. As you inhale, step forward with your right foot, about the length of your leg. Keep your feet even with your hips, your legs straight with a slight bend in your knees, and your weight placed evenly from front leg to back. Keep your feet flat on the floor and both hipbones facing forward. Rest your right hand lightly on your right thigh while your left arm rests by your side.

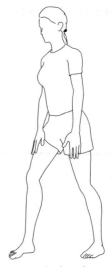

**Inhale and step your right foot forward, about a leg's length. Be sure to keep your balance.**

3. Lift your left arm by your ear as you bend your right knee over your right ankle, leading with your chest, inhaling as you go. Pause here to s-t-r-e-t-c-h.

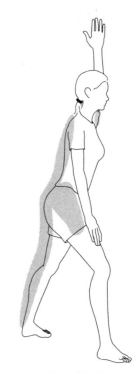

**Pause here to stretch, and feel it in your hip, back, and left arm.**

4. Exhale, straighten your right leg, and move your arm down by your side. Repeat this movement four times, remembering envelope breathing. As you move, keep your upper body relaxed to prevent tension in your back, shoulders, and neck.

5. Step your right foot back to the starting position, check your balance, and then step your left foot forward as you inhale, your left hand on your left thigh, your right arm at your side. Repeat the movements four times on this side of your body. Return to the starting position to pause, check your balance, and relax your breath.

## Hamstring Stretch (Chapter 2)

1. Lie on your back, your knees bent, with your feet on the floor, even with and a comfortable distance away from your hips. Rest your arms beside your body. Draw your knees toward your chest as you exhale.

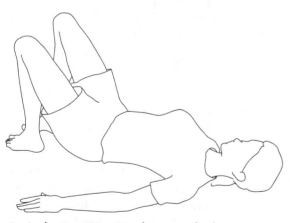

Begin the Hamstring Stretch on your back, your arms at your sides, your feet hip-width apart on the floor.

2. Lift your feet toward the ceiling as you inhale deeply, straightening your legs and raising your arms back over your head toward the floor behind you. You can keep a bend in your knees if your hamstrings are tight. Keep your lower back flat on the floor.

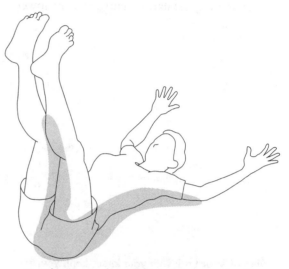

Stretch out your hamstrings while remembering to breathe.

3. Bend your knees toward your chest, hands on your knees, curling up like a ball as you exhale. Keep your head on the floor.

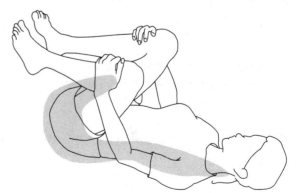

Use your hands on your knees to deepen the stretch.

4. Repeat steps 2 and 3 three more times, moving while you breathe, and then hold your knees and rest.

# Spinal Roll (Chapter 8)

1. Lie on your back, knees bent, feet placed a comfortable distance from your buttocks and hip-width apart. Rest your arms by your sides. Take a deep breath, and exhale as you roll your tailbone to your nose, flattening the natural curve at your lower back.

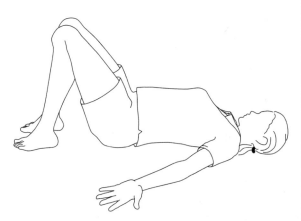

*Lying on your back with your knees bent, your feet hip-width apart, your arms by your sides, show no natural curve at your lower back.*

2. Inhale with your tailbone tucked, and slowly lift your hips as you exhale. With your hips lifted, take in a deep breath.

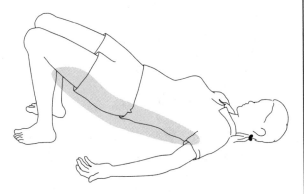

*Lie on your back, your feet hip-width apart and parallel, your arms by sides, and your hips lifted.*

3. As you exhale, slowly lower your spine to the floor one vertebrae at a time until your whole spine is resting on the floor. Relax for a few moments, feeling the natural curve at your lower back.

4. Repeat steps 1 through 3 three more times.

# Knee Press (Chapter 8)

1. Lie on your back on a comfortable surface (but not your bed). Inhale deeply. As you exhale, draw one knee toward your chest. Inhale again, and with the next exhale, draw your other knee toward your chest. Place your hands lightly on each knee. Tuck your chin toward your chest while keeping your head on the floor.

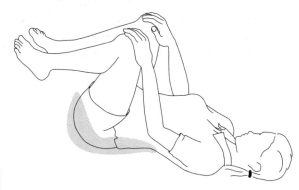

*Lying on your back, bend your knees toward your chest, with one hand on each knee and your elbows bent.*

2. Move your thighs away from your chest as you inhale and straighten your arms. Keep your hands on your knees. Move your thighs toward your chest, bending your elbows as you exhale. Do not pull or force your legs toward your chest. Practice these movements eight times.

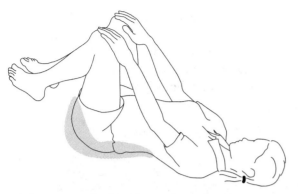

Lying on your back with your knees bent, rest one hand on each knee and extended and straighten your arms.

3. With your head resting on the floor, grasp your arms around your knees to form your body into a ball. Hold on to your hand, wrist, or forearm as you draw your knees toward your chest. Rest your head on the floor. Take one deep, full breath in this position. Inhale, and as you exhale, bring your nose toward your knees, engaging your abdominal muscles as you move.

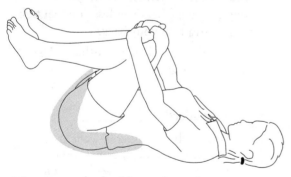

Lying on your back with your knees bent, wrap your arms around your legs, keeping your head on the floor.

4. Lower your upper back to the floor and relax your shoulders as you inhale. Repeat these movements two more times, then rest with your hands on your knees for a few moments.

## Heels Over Head Stretch (Chapter 6)

1. Lie on your right side, close to a wall, with your knees bent toward your chest. Scoot your hips so your feet and buttocks touch the wall.

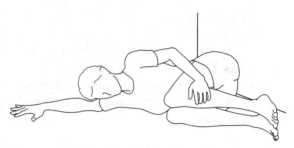

Lie on your right side with your knees bent, your feet and buttocks touching the wall.

2. Roll to the left, swinging your legs up the wall. Open your arms from your shoulders out to the sides, palms up. If you feel tension in the backs of your legs, turn your legs slightly in and release any tightness in your knees.

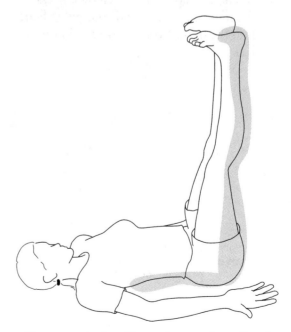

Lie on your back, with your legs up the wall and your arms stretched out.

3. Relax into the stretch and breathe deeply, holding the position at least 5 minutes. Your breathing should become slow and deep as you hold the stretch, relieving stress and relaxing muscles in your forehead, eyes, jaw, and tongue.

4. Come out of the stretch, retracing the steps you took to move into it. Bend your knees, roll to your side, and use your strong arms to move to your hands and knees. Place one foot on the floor, with your knee bent, and hold on to a chair or the wall for support as you raise your body to standing.

## Reclining Fork (Chapter 8)

1. Lie on your belly, your forehead touching the floor. Place your forearms and palms flat on the floor so your arms are in a 90-degree position. Your elbows should line up with your shoulders, and your hands should line up with your elbows. Press the tops of your feet and your pubic bone into the floor. Notice how your lower back feels.

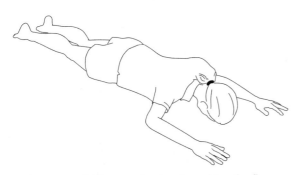

Lie on your belly, your forehead touching the floor, your arms in a box position with your forearms and palms flat on the floor.

2. As you exhale, slowly lift your chest off the floor, using your back muscles rather than your hands. Keep your mind on how your lower back feels as you lift your chest. Raise your chin slightly.

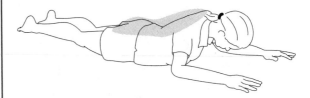

Lie on your belly with your palms flat on the floor, your arms in a box position with your forearms and palms flat on the floor and your chest lifted.

3. Hold the stretch as you inhale. Lower your chest to the floor as you exhale. Inhale with your chest on the floor. Lift your chest again as you exhale, hold your chest up as you inhale, and lower your chest as you exhale. Repeat these movements two more times. Hold the stretch with your chest lifted off the floor for three breaths. Remember not to place any weight in your hands unless you feel tightness or strain in your back.

4. Release the stretch as you exhale. Rest and notice the results.

**Flex Alert!**

If you feel any tension in your lower back after you practice the Reclining Fork, move into the Knee Press from Chapter 8.

# Stretching Resources

Maybe you're motivated to stretch; however, you might need the support of a teacher or helpful supplies to enjoy your stretching experience. There's no substitute for a good teacher to help design a program to meet your unique needs. Your teacher may also support and guide you as you learn more about your body. Steadiness and comfort are key principles that need to be in place for you to make the most of your stretching routine. Providing yourself with the supplies outlined in this guide will serve to make your experience enjoyable and safe.

## Stretching Professionals

**Bob and Jean Anderson**
Stretching Inc.
PO Box 767
Palmer Lake, CO 80133
1-800-333-1307
www.stretching.com

**Janis Bowersox**
Owner and Registered Yoga Teacher
Yoga for Everybody, LLC
27 Unquowa Road
Fairfield, CT 06824
203-254-YOGA (203-254-9642)
www.yoga4everybody.net

**Yoga for You**
Trish Deignan, CYI, Physical Therapist Asst.
Laguna Beach, CA 92651
949-310-9343

**Shoban Richard Faulds**
Kripalu Center for Yoga and Health
PO Box 309
Stockbridge, MA 01262

**Jennifer Gilley**
Registered Yoga Instructor, Kripalu certified,
RYT Yoga Alliance
860-379-5481
jennifergilley@sbcglobal.net

**Jennifer Legault**
Certified Perinatal Support Specialist
Prenatal Yoga Instructor
Beautifully Birthed Certified
Labor Support Services
Laguna Beach, CA
949-981-2283
jennifer@beautifullybirthed.com
www.beautifullybirthed.com

**Aaron L. Mattes, MS, RKT, LMT**
*Active Isolated Stretching: The Mattes Method*,
leader of "Active Isolated Stretching" seminars
PO Box 17217
Sarasota, FL 34276
941-922-1939
stretchingusa@comcast.net
www.stretchingusa.com

**Sara Pearson, M.A.**
Registered Yoga Instructor
949-375-4375
kjpsfp@aol.com

**Anita White-Barbero**
"Renew Your Health"; designer of "Strength
and Spirit" fitness class; fitness consultant
barberoent@optonline.net
www.renewwithanita.com

**Barbara Templeton**
*The Complete Idiot's Guide to Stretching* Online
www.cigstretching.com

**Mark Whitwell**
*Yoga of Heart: The Healing Power of
Intimate Connection*
www.heartofyoga.com

**Juris Zinbergs**
316 Poplar Street, #B
Laguna Beach, CA 92651
sradha3@mac.com

**Diana Pollaro, RYT-500**
Certified Kripalu Professional Level Yoga
Teacher
Certified Prenatal Yoga Teacher
diana@yogaontherun.com
www.yogaontherun.com

# Stretching Supplies

**Playground Ball**
These inexpensive 5-inch-diameter rubber playground balls can be found at your local sporting goods store. You can also purchase them directly from the manufacturer online at www.mikasasports.com.

**Blankets, Straps, Bolsters, and Mats**
Hugger-Mugger Yoga Products
3937 South 500 West
Salt Lake City, UT 84123
1-800-473-4888
www.huggermugger.com

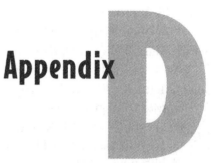

**Appendix D**

# Find Out More

Explore stretches to address your unique needs with the following books and articles. Have fun experimenting with advanced stretches, or nurture an area of your body that needs special attention. Discover the joy of breathing deeply into your stretches, and learn more about your amazing body!

## Books and Articles

Anderson, Bob, and Jean Anderson. *Stretching*. Bolinas, CA: Shelter Publications, 2000.

Balaskas, Janet. *Preparing for Birth with Yoga*. London: Element Books, 1994.

Calais-Germain, Blandine. *Anatomy of Movement*. Seattle: Eastland Press, 1991.

Farhi, Donna. *The Breathing Book*. New York: Henry Holt and Company, 1996.

Faulds, Richard, and Senior Teaching Staff KCYH. *Kripalu Yoga: A Guide to Practice on and off the Mat*. New York: Bantam Dell, 2006.

Jordan, Sandra. *Yoga for Pregnancy*. New York: St. Martin's Press, 1987.

Kraftsow, Gary. *Yoga for Wellness*. New York: Penguin Group, 1999.

Mohan, A. G. *Yoga for Body, Breath and Mind*. Boston: Shambhala Publications, 2002.

Mohan, A. G., and Indra. *Yoga Therapy*. Boston: Shambhala Publications, 2004.

Ramaswami, Srivatsa. *The Complete Book of Vinyasa Yoga*. New York: Marlowe & Company, 2005.

Saraswati, Swami Satyananda. *Asana Pranayama Mudra Bandha*. Bihar, India: Bihar School of Yoga, 1999.

Scaravelli, Vanda. *Awakening the Spine*. San Francisco: HarperCollins, 1991.

Schatz, Mary Pullig, M.D. *Back Care Basics*. Berkeley: Rodmell Press, 1992.

Solan, Matthew. "Easy Rider," *Yoga Journal Magazine*, August 2006.

Uppgaard, Robert O., D.D.S. *Taking Control of TMJ*. Oakland: New Harbinger Publications, 1999.

Whitwell, Mark. *Yoga of Heart: The Healing Power of Intimate Connection*. New York: Lantern Books, 2004.

# Websites

**www.cigstretching.com**
Check out *The Complete Idiot's Guide to Stretching Illustrated* blog to keep up to date with Jamie and Barbara Templeton, the authors of *The Complete Idiot's Guide to Stretching Illustrated*.

**www.breathingyoga.com**
Find out what's going on at Breathing Yoga.

**www.vinyasakrama.com**
Meet my teacher, the legendary Srivatsa Ramaswami, and explore his events, photos, and chants.

**www.huggermugger.com**
Check out the ultimate gear provider for mind, body, and spirit.

**www.mayoclinic.com**
Visit the renowned Mayo Clinic online and learn all you need to know to stay healthy, strong, and flexible.

**www.mikasasports.com**
Mikasa provides equipment for all your favorite sports.

**www.nia.nih.gov**
Go to the National Institute on Aging to review the latest research on health issues facing you as you mature.

**www.stretch.com**
Meet Carol Dickman, a stretching professional, and enjoy stretches for humans and pets.

**www.stretching.com**
The official website for Bob and Jean Anderson's book *Stretching*.

**www.stretchingusa.com**
Meet Aaron Mattes and learn more about Active Isolated Stretching.

**www.viniyoga.com**
Learn therapuetic stretches from Gary Kraftsow.

**www.walking.about.com**
Discover how walking can keep you healthy and strong.

**www.yogajournal.com**
*Yoga Journal* magazine's offical website, where you can find all you need to know about yoga.

# Index

## A

adductors, 54-55
adhesive capsulitis, 92
aerobic activities, 124
    Kneeling Hip Flexor, 128-129
    One Leg Up, One Leg Down, 127
    Pyramid, 125-126
    Standing Quadriceps, 129-130
    Triangle Stretch with Moving Leg, 130-131
A Frame, 85-86
    PMS (premenstrual
      syndrome), 160-161
    swimming, 134-135
alignment, stretching benefits, 7-8
anatomy, 11-12
Ankle Alive, swimming, 136-137
Ankle Circles, 59-60, 141
Ankle Rolls, pregnancy, 170
Ankles Alive, 58-59
arms, Prayer, 36-37
Asymmetrical Hip, cycling, 133

## B

Back Arch, menopause, 171
backs
    discomforts, 108
      arch and curl, 109-110
      Heels Over Head, 113

Knee as Handle, 112-113
    Knee Press, 110-111
    relaxing on ball, 108-109
    sciatica, 114-118
    Z stretch, 111-112
strengtheners, 119
    Dragon's Tail, 121
    Reclining Fork, 120-121
    Spinal Roll, 119-120
top-of-the body stretches
    Figure Eight, 33-34
    Pretzel, 32-33
    Sun and Earth, 30-31
balance exercises
    Part 1, 156
    Part 2, 157
    stretching benefits, 7-8
base
    basics, 41-42
    calves, 56
      Ankle Circles, 59-60
      Ankles Alive, 58-59
      Double Knee Bends, 60-61
      On Your Toes, 56-57
      Toe Tinglers, 57-58
    feet, 56
      Ankle Circles, 59-60
      Ankles Alive, 58-59
      Double Knee Bends, 60-61
      On Your Toes, 56-57
      Toe Tinglers, 57-58

hips, 42
    Diamond, 42-43
    Number 4, 43-45
    Reclining Hip Flexor, 46
    Runner's stretch, 45-46
    Standing Hip Flexor, 46-48
knees, 56
    Ankle Circles, 59-60
    Ankles Alive, 58-59
    Double Knee Bends, 60-61
    On Your Toes, 56-57
    Toe Tinglers, 57-58
legs, 48
    Hamstring Stretch with Hands, 52-53
    Inner Thigh, 54
    Kneeling Quadriceps, 50-51
    Outer Thigh, 55
    Pyramid, 49-50
    Standing Quadriceps, 51-52
bicycling legs, 17-18
bodies
    anatomy basics, 11-12
    listening to, 15-16
    lower
        base basics, 41-42
        calves, 56-61
        feet, 56-61
        hips, 42-48
        knees, 56-61
        legs, 48-55
    mindful stretching, 13
    regular routine, 12-13
    top-of-the body stretches
        back, 30-34
        chest, 34-37
        hands, 37-39
        head, 26-29
        shoulders, 30-33
        wrists, 37-39
    warming up, 16-17
        bicycling legs, 17-18
        gentle twist, 18-19
        hamstring stretch, 20-21
        morning stretch, 17
        spinal roll, 19-20

whole body stretches
    gentle stretches, 64-71
    strong stretches, 71-79
bones, structure, 11
Bowl stretch, CTS (carpal
  tunnel syndrome), 100
breathing, 14-15
burnout, 176

## C

calves, 56
    Ankle Circles, 59-60
    Ankles Alive, 58-59
    Double Knee Bends, 60-61
    On Your Toes, 56-57
    Toe Tinglers, 57-58
carpal tunnel syndrome (CTS), 96
    Bowl stretch, 100
    Entire Front stretch, 96-97
    Pretzel, 97-98
    Reclining Fork, 99
cartilage, 12
Chest Expander, 34-35
chests, top-of-the body stretches
    Chest Expander, 34-35
    Prayer, 36-37
    Relaxing Chest Opener, 34
chronic tension, necks, 89
    Kneeling Neck, 90-91
    Seated Neck, 89-90
contradictions, 89
CTS (carpal tunnel syndrome), 96
    Bowl stretch, 100
    Entire Front stretch, 96-97
    Pretzel, 97-98
    Reclining Fork, 99
cycling, 131
    Asymmetrical Hip, 133
    Z stretch, 132

## D

Deep Breathing, TMJD (Temporomandibular Joint Disorder), 87-88
Diamond, 42-43, 136
discomforts, 16
    backs, 108
        arch and curl, 109-110
        Heels Over Head, 113
        Knee as Handle, 112-113
        Knee Press, 110-111
        relaxing on ball, 108-109
        sciatica, 114-118
        strengtheners, 119-121
        Z stretch, 111-112
    CTS (carpal tunnel syndrome), 96
        Bowl stretch, 100
        Entire Front stretch, 96-97
        Pretzel, 97-98
        Reclining Fork, 99
    headaches, 84
        A Frame, 85-86
        Heels Over Head, 84-85
    hips, 101
        Outer Thigh, 104-105
        Reclining Hip Flexor, 102
        Single Knee Bends, 101-102
        Triangle, 103
    knees, 101
        Outer Thigh, 104-105
        Reclining Hip Flexor, 102
        Single Knee Bends, 101-102
        Triangle, 103
    neck tension, 89
        Kneeling Neck, 90-91
        Seated Neck, 89-90
    shoulders, 91-92
        Sun and Earth, 93
        Supine Shoulder, 92
    TMJD (Temporomandibular Joint Disorder), 87
        Deep Breathing, 87-88
        Relax Your Jaw, 88
        Stretch Your Jaw, 88-89
Double Knee Bends, 60-61
Dragon's Tail, strengthening back, 121
dynamic stretching, 13-14

## E

Eagle Eye, 26-27
edge, 15
elasticity, anatomy basics, 11-12
Entire Front stretch, CTS (carpal tunnel syndrome), 96-97
envelope breathing, 15
Eye Push-Ups, 28
eyes
    Eagle Eye, 26-27
    Eye Push-Ups, 28

## F

fascia, 12
feet, 56
    Ankle Circles, 59-60
    Ankles Alive, 58-59
    Double Knee Bends, 60-61
    On Your Toes, 56-57
    Toe Tinglers, 57-58
Figure Eight, 33-34
Finger Wrap, 37-38
flat backs, 69
flexibility
    mindful of body, 13
    regular routine, 12-13
frozen shoulder, 92
Full Back
    gentle, 70-71
    strong, 77-79

## G

Gentle Full Back, 70-71
Gentle Half Back, 68-69
Gentle Side, 65-67
Gentle Twist, 67-68
golf, 139
    Ankle Circles, 141
    Knee Press, 146
    Lunging Forward and Back, 148
    Puppy Stretch, 144

Reclining Twist, 142
Seated Neck, 140
Standing Chest, 147
Standing Quadriceps, 145
Standing Squat, 143
Wrist Wave, 139-140
gravity, reversing cures, 84
    A Frame, 85-86
    Heels Over Head, 84-85

## H

Half Back
    gentle, 68-69
    strong, 76-77
hamstrings, warming up, 20-21
Hamstring Stretch with Hands, 52-53
hands
    Prayer, 36-37
    top-of-the body stretches, 37
        Finger Wrap, 37-38
        Wrist Circles, 38-39
        Wrist Waves, 38
headaches, reverse gravity cures, 84
    A Frame, 85-86
    Heels Over Head, 84-85
heads, top-of-the body stretches, 26
    Eagle Eye, 26-27
    Eye Push-Ups, 28
    Jolly Jaws, 29
healing benefits, 7
Heels Over Head, 84-85
    back discomfort, 113
    menopause, 174
hiking, 124
    Kneeling Hip Flexor, 128-129
    One Leg Up, One Leg Down, 127
    Pyramid, 125-126
    Standing Quadriceps, 129-130
    Triangle Stretch with Moving Leg, 130-131
hip flexors, 41-42
hip rotators, 41-42
hips, 42
    Diamond, 42-43

discomforts, 101
    Outer Thigh, 104-105
    Reclining Hip Flexor, 102
    Single Knee Bends, 101-102
    Triangle, 103
Number 4, 43-45
Reclining Hip Flexor, 46
Runner's stretch, 45-46
Standing Hip Flexor, 46-48

## I-J

iliotibial (IT) bands, 55
Inner Thigh, 54
intercostal muscles, 30
IT (iliotibial) bands, 55
jaws, Jolly Jaws, 29
Jolly Jaws, 29
Journal of the American Medical Association, The, 114
J stretch, menopause, 175

## K

Knee as Handle, back discomfort, 112-113
Kneeling Hip Flexor, aerobic sports, 128-129
Kneeling Neck, 90-91
Kneeling Quadriceps, 50-51
Knee Presses
    back discomfort, 110-111
    golf and tennis, 146
    menopause, 172-173
knees, 56
    Ankle Circles, 59-60
    Ankles Alive, 58-59
    discomforts, 101
        Outer Thigh, 104-105
        Reclining Hip Flexor, 102
        Single Knee Bends, 101-102
        Triangle, 103
    Double Knee Bends, 60-61
    On Your Toes, 56-57
    Toe Tinglers, 57-58

# L

lactic acids, 124
ladies
    Ankle Rolls, 170
    menopause, 171
        Back Arch, 171
        Heels Over Head, 174
        J stretch, 175
        Knee Press, 172-173
    PMS (premenstrual syndrome), 160
        A Frame, 160-161
        Leap Frog, 162
        Reclining Number 4, 163
    pregnancy, 164
        Meditative, 169
        Modified Twist, 165-166
        Partner Squat, 168
        Reclining Frog, 164-165
        Right Angle at Wall, 167
    stress, 176
        Reclining Diamond, 178
        Reclining Twist, 179
        Z stretch, 176-177
Leap Frog stretch, PMS (premenstrual syndrome), 162
legs, 48
    bicycling, 17-18
    Hamstring Stretch with Hands, 52-53
    Inner Thigh, 54
    Kneeling Quadriceps, 50-51
    Outer Thigh, 55
    Pyramid, 49-50
    Standing Quadriceps, 51-52
ligaments, 12
lower body stretches
    base basics, 41-42
    calves, 56
        Ankle Circles, 59-60
        Ankles Alive, 58-59
        Double Knee Bends, 60-61
        On Your Toes, 56-57
        Toe Tinglers, 57-58
    feet, 56
        Ankle Circles, 59-60
        Ankles Alive, 58-59
        Double Knee Bends, 60-61
        On Your Toes, 56-57
        Toe Tinglers, 57-58
    hips, 42
        Diamond, 42-43
        Number 4, 43-45
        Reclining Hip Flexor, 46
        Runner's stretch, 45-46
        Standing Hip Flexor, 46-48
    knees, 56
        Ankle Circles, 59-60
        Ankles Alive, 58-59
        Double Knee Bends, 60-61
        On Your Toes, 56-57
        Toe Tinglers, 57-58
    legs, 48
        Hamstring Stretch with Hands, 52-53
        Inner Thigh, 54
        Kneeling Quadriceps, 50-51
        Outer Thigh, 55
        Pyramid, 49-50
        Standing Quadriceps, 51-52
Lunging Forward and Back, golf and tennis, 148

# M

Meditative, pregnancy, 169
meniscus, 56
menopause, 171
    Back Arch, 171
    Heels Over Head, 174
    J stretch, 175
    Knee Press, 172-173
misalignments, structural, 8
Modified Twist stretch, pregnancy, 165-166
morning stretches, 17
muscles, 12
    intercostal, 30
    piriformis, 114
    psoas, 46
musculoskeletal conditions, 41-42

## N-O

necks, tension, 89
    Kneeling Neck, 90-91
    Seated Neck, 89-90
Number 4, 43-45
One Leg Up, One Leg Down, 115-116, 127
On Your Toes, 56-57
osteoarthritis, 101
Outer Thigh, 55, 104-105, 118

## P

pains, 16
Partner Squat, pregnancy, 168
pelvis, 12
piriformis muscles, 114
PMS (premenstrual syndrome), 160
    A Frame, 160-161
    Leap Frog, 162
    Reclining Number 4, 163
Prayer stretch, 36-37
pregnancies, 164
    Ankle Rolls, 170
    Meditative, 169
    Modified Twist, 165-166
    Partner Squat, 168
    Reclining Frog, 164-165
    Right Angle at Wall, 167
premenstrual syndrome (PMS), 160
    A Frame, 160-161
    Leap Frog, 162
    Reclining Number 4, 163
Pretzel, 32-33
    CTS (carpal tunnel syndrome), 97-98
    swimming, 138-139
proprioception stretching, 14
psoas muscles, 46
Puppy Stretch, golf and tennis, 144
Pyramid, 49-50, 125-126

## Q-R

quadriceps, 48
range of motion, 6, 19
Receiving, 64-65
Reclining Diamond, women's stress, 178
Reclining Fork
    CTS (carpal tunnel syndrome), 99
    strengthening back, 120-121
Reclining Frog, pregnancy, 164-165
Reclining Hip Flexor, 46, 102
Reclining Number 4, PMS (premenstrual syndrome), 163
Reclining Right Angle, 116
Reclining Twist
    golf and tennis, 142
    women's stress, 179
Relaxing Chest Opener, 34
Relax Your Jaw stretch, TMJD (Temporomandibular Joint Disorder), 88
reverse gravity cures, headaches, 84
    A Frame, 85-86
    Heels Over Head, 84-85
Right Angle at Wall, pregnancy, 167
routines, maintaining flexibility, 12-13
Runner's stretch, 45-46
running, 124
    Kneeling Hip Flexor, 128-129
    One Leg Up, One Leg Down, 127
    Pyramid, 125-126
    Standing Quadriceps, 129-130
    Triangle Stretch with Moving Leg, 130-131

## S

sacrums, 12, 109
sciatica, back discomfort, 114
    One Leg Up, One Leg Down, 115-116
    Outer Thigh, 118
    Reclining Right Angle, 116
    Seated Sciatic, 114-115
    Standing Right Angle, 116-117
Seated Chest Expander, senior seated stretches, 152-153

Seated Forward Bend, senior seated stretches, 155
Seated Neck, 89-90, 140
Seated Sciatic, 114-115
seated stretches, seniors, 152
    Seated Chest Expander, 152-153
    Seated Forward Bend, 155
    Seated Twist, 154
Seated Twist, senior seated stretches, 154
seniors
    seated stretches, 152
        Seated Chest Expander, 152-153
        Seated Forward Bend, 155
        Seated Twist, 154
    standing stretches, 156
        Part 1 balance exercise, 156
        Part 2 balance exercise, 157
Shoulder and Chest Expander, 71-72
shoulder girdles, 12
shoulders
    sore, 91-92
        Sun and Earth, 93
        Supine Shoulder, 92
    top-of-the body stretches
        Pretzel, 32-33
        Sun and Earth, 30-31
Side stretches
    gentle, 65-67
    strong, 73-74
Single Knee Bends, 101-102
skeletons, 11
Spinal Rolls
    strengthening back, 119-120
    warming up, 19-20
spines, 12
    gentle twists, 18-19
    rolls, 19-20
sports
    aerobic activities, 124
        Kneeling Hip Flexor, 128-129
        One Leg Up, One Leg Down, 127
        Pyramid, 125-126
        Standing Quadriceps, 129-130
        Triangle Stretch with Moving Leg, 130-131
    cycling, 131
        Asymmetrical Hip, 133
        Z stretch, 132

golf, 139
    Ankle Circles, 141
    Knee Press, 146
    Lunging Forward and Back, 148
    Puppy Stretch, 144
    Reclining Twist, 142
    Seated Neck, 140
    Standing Chest, 147
    Standing Quadriceps, 145
    Standing Squat, 143
    Wrist Wave, 139-140
stretching basics, 124
swimming, 134
    A Frame, 134-135
    Ankle Alive, 136-137
    Diamond, 136
    Pretzel, 138-139
tennis, 139
    Ankle Circles, 141
    Knee Press, 146
    Lunging Forward and Back, 148
    Puppy Stretch, 144
    Reclining Twist, 142
    Seated Neck, 140
    Standing Chest, 147
    Standing Quadriceps, 145
    Standing Squat, 143
    Wrist Wave, 139-140
Standing Chest stretch, golf and tennis, 147
Standing Hip Flexor, 46-48
Standing Quadriceps, 51-52
    aerobic sports, 129-130
    golf and tennis, 145
Standing Right Angle, 116-117
Standing Squat, golf and tennis, 143
standing stretches, seniors, 156
    Part 1 balance exercise, 156
    Part 2 balance exercise, 157
static stretching, 13-14
sternum, 144
strengthening backs, 119
    Dragon's Tail, 121
    Reclining Fork, 120-121
    Spinal Roll, 119-120

stress, women, 176
  Reclining Diamond, 178
  Reclining Twist, 179
  Z stretch, 176-177
stretching
  animals, 5
  anyone can stretch, 8-9
  babies, 5
  benefits, 6
    alignment and balance, 7-8
    healing, 7
    healthful habits, 6-7
    making time in your schedule, 7
  breathing, 14-15
  defined, 5-6
  for athletes, 8
  listening to body, 15-16
  types, 13-14
  warming up, 16-17
    bicycling legs, 17-18
    gentle twist, 18-19
    hamstring stretch, 20-21
    morning stretch, 17
    spinal roll, 19-20
Stretch Your Jaw, TMJD (Temporomandibular Joint Disorder), 88-89
Strong Full Back, 77-79
Strong Half Back, 76-77
Strong Side, 73-74
Strong Twist, 74-76
structural misalignment, 8
Sun and Earth routine, 30-31
Sun and Earth, 93
Supine Shoulder, 92
swimming, 134
  Ankle Alive, 136-137
  Diamond, 136
  A Frame, 134-135
  Pretzel, 138-139
synovial fluids, 16

**T**

temporal bones, 87
Temporomandibular Joint Disorder (TMJD), 87
  Deep Breathing, 87-88
  Relax Your Jaw, 88
  Stretch Your Jaw, 88-89
tendons, 12
tennis, 139
  Ankle Circles, 141
  Knee Press, 146
  Lunging Forward and Back, 148
  Puppy Stretch, 144
  Reclining Twist, 142
  Seated Neck, 140
  Standing Chest, 147
  Standing Quadriceps, 145
  Standing Squat, 143
  Wrist Wave, 139-140
tension, necks, 89
  Kneeling Neck, 90-91
  Seated Neck, 89-90
thighs
  Inner, 54
  Outer, 55
TMJD (Temporomandibular Joint Disorder), 87
  Deep Breathing, 87-88
  Relax Your Jaw, 88
  Stretch Your Jaw, 88-89
toes
  On Your Toes, 56-57
  Toe Tinglers, 57-58
Toe Tinglers, 57-58
top-of-the body stretches
  back
    Figure Eight, 33-34
    Pretzel, 32-33
    Sun and Earth, 30-31
  chest
    Chest Expander, 34-35
    Prayer, 36-37
    Relaxing Chest Opener, 34

hands, 37
    Finger Wrap, 37-38
    Wrist Circles, 38-39
    Wrist Waves, 38
head, 26
    Eagle Eye, 26-27
    Eye Push-Ups, 28
    Jolly Jaws, 29
shoulders
    Pretzel, 32-33
    Sun and Earth, 30-31
wrists, 37
    Finger Wrap, 37-38
    Wrist Circles, 38-39
    Wrist Waves, 38
treatment plans
    backs, 108
        arch and curl, 109-110
        Heels Over Head, 113
        Knee as Handle, 112-113
        Knee Press, 110-111
        relaxing on ball, 108-109
        sciatica, 114-118
        strengtheners, 119-121
        Z stretch, 111-112
    CTS (carpal tunnel syndrome), 96
        Bowl stretch, 100
        Entire Front stretch, 96-97
        Pretzel, 97-98
        Reclining Fork, 99
    headaches, 84
        A Frame, 85-86
        Heels Over Head, 84-85
    hips, 101
        Outer Thigh, 104-105
        Reclining Hip Flexor, 102
        Single Knee Bends, 101-102
        Triangle, 103
    knees, 101
        Outer Thigh, 104-105
        Reclining Hip Flexor, 102
        Single Knee Bends, 101-102
        Triangle, 103
    neck tension, 89
        Kneeling Neck, 90-91
        Seated Neck, 89-90

shoulders, 91-92
    Sun and Earth, 93
    Supine Shoulder, 92
TMJD (Temporomandibular Joint Disorder), 87
Deep Breathing, 87-88
Relax Your Jaw, 88
Stretch Your Jaw, 88-89
Triangle, 103
Triangle Stretch with Moving Leg, aerobic sports, 130-131
twists, warming up, 18-19
Twist
    gentle, 67-68
    strong, 74-76

## U

upper bodies
    back
        Figure Eight, 33-34
        Pretzel, 32-33
        Sun and Earth, 30-31
    chest
        Chest Expander, 34-35
        Prayer, 36-37
        Relaxing Chest Opener, 34
    hands, 37
        Finger Wrap, 37-38
        Wrist Circles, 38-39
        Wrist Waves, 38
    head, 26
        Eagle Eye, 26-27
        Eye Push-Ups, 28
        Jolly Jaws, 29
    shoulders
        Pretzel, 32-33
        Sun and Earth, 30-31
    wrists, 37
        Finger Wrap, 37-38
        Wrist Circles, 38-39
        Wrist Waves, 38

# W

walking, 124
  Kneeling Hip Flexor stretch, 128-129
  One Leg Up, One Leg Down stretch, 127
  Pyramid stretch, 125-126
  Standing Quadriceps stretch, 129-130
  Triangle Stretch with Moving Leg stretch, 130-131
warm ups, 16-17
  bicycling legs, 17-18
  gentle twist, 18-19
  hamstring stretch, 20-21
  morning stretch, 17
  spinal roll, 19-20
whole body
  gentle stretches, 64
    Gentle Full Back, 70-71
    Gentle Half Back, 68-69
    Gentle Side, 65-67
    Gentle Twist, 67-68
    Receiving, 64-65
  strong stretches, 71
    Shoulder and Chest Expander, 71-72
    Strong Full Back, 77-79
    Strong Half Back, 76-77
    Strong Side, 73-74
    Strong Twist, 74-76
women
  menopause, 171
    Back Arch, 171
    Heels Over Head, 174
    J stretch, 175
    Knee Press, 172-173
  PMS (premenstrual syndrome), 160
    A Frame, 160-161
    Leap Frog, 162
    Reclining Number 4, 163
  pregnancy, 164
    Ankle Rolls, 170
    Meditative, 169
    Modified Twist, 165-166
    Partner Squat, 168
    Reclining Frog, 164-165
    Right Angle at Wall, 167

  stress, 176
    Reclining Diamond, 178
    Reclining Twist, 179
    Z stretch, 176-177
Wrist Circles, 38-39
wrists, top-of-the body stretches, 37
  Finger Wrap, 37-38
  Wrist Circles, 38-39
  Wrist Waves, 38
Wrist Waves, 38, 139-140

# X-Y-Z

Z stretch
  back discomfort, 111-112
  cycling, 132
  women's stress, 176-177

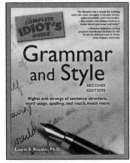
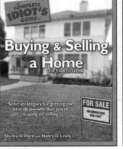
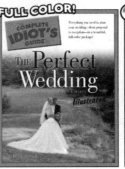
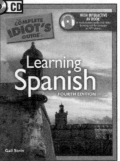
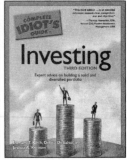
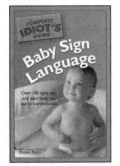
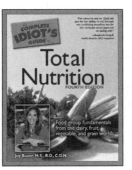
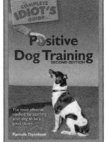
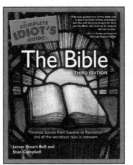
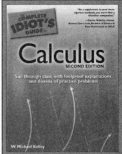
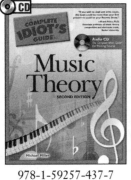
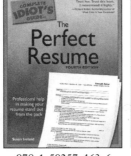
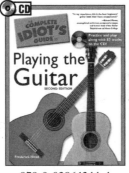
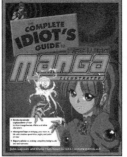
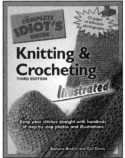
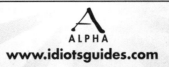